D1231789

HOSPITAL INFORMATION SYSTEMS

BIOMEDICAL ENGINEERING

A Series of Monographs

SERIES EDITOR

GEORGE A. BEKEY

University of Southern California
Los Angeles, California

volume 1   Hospital Information Systems
Edited by George A. Bekey
and Morton D. Schwartz

Other volumes in preparation.

HOSPITAL INFORMATION SYSTEMS

EDITED BY

George A. Bekey and Morton D. Schwartz

University of Southern California
Los Angeles, California

California State College
Long Beach, California

MARCEL DEKKER, INC., New York   1972

COPYRIGHT © 1972 by MARCEL DEKKER, INC.

MARCEL DEKKER, INC.

95 Madison Avenue, New York, New York 10016

LIBRARY OF CONGRESS CATALOG
CARD NUMBER: 70-190097

ISBN 0-8247-1034-7

Printed in the United States of America

Preface

The day to day operation of a modern hospital involves the handling of vast quantities of information. In view of the multiple functions of a hospital, the data involved in this information flow is highly variable in content, format, and importance. Data arising from the clinical laboratories, pharmacy orders, x-ray results, or on-line results in an intensive care unit may be essential in the treatment of disease and the saving of lives. Yet, alongside with such direct patient management data, the hospital involves a multiplicity of indirect information concerning its hotel-like activities, including bed inventories, linen supplies, meal planning, and the delivery of a multitude of services to the wards. Finally, the business office of the hospital must maintain accounting and provide billing for services for both in-patients and out-patients, in view of an array of complex insurance and government requirements.

To keep up with this explosion in information, hospitals are turning increasingly to the use of automatic computer-based methods of information storage, handling, and retrieval. Collectively, we refer to such systems as Hospital Information Systems. We define a hospital information system as a high-speed, computer-controlled, multi-station, authorized-access, information flow network for the hospital. It has both business office and patient care subsystems, and its function is to speed and simplify the handling of both administrative and medical information. The hospital staff has access to the system through the use of data terminals located

at nursing stations and other strategic points in the various
departments and service areas.

The hospital information system stores, retrieves,
routes, monitors, sorts, and verifies the flow of information.
It can be designed to provide patient medical histories,
current medical records, statistical summaries, and legal
records. It can schedule medical services and maintain
inventory control of beds and supplies. As a result of this
complex and versatile array of functions, it is evident that
hospital information systems can not only automate data
handling within the hospital but can provide a completely new
set of management techniques for the modern hospital.

This book is an overview of the state of the art in
hospital information systems. It is based on presentations
made in short courses held at the University of Southern
California each summer since 1969. The various chapters in
the book highlight the major problems in the implementation
of hospital information systems and their applications in such
areas as the clinical laboratory, the hospital ward, the intensive care unit, the pharmacy, the multi-test screening
center, and the business office. Both hardware and software
aspects of hospital information systems are discussed, in
order to make it possible to assess the influence of such
systems on the management of the hospital, on the costs of
health care, and on the quality of medical service.

The book should be of interest to professional personnel
concerned with modern trends in the delivery of health care,
including biomedical engineers, architects, data processing
specialists, hospital administrators, physicians, and paramedical personnel. It is our hope that it will assist hospital
staff members planning the installation of new information
systems, by providing them with a record of both success
stories and difficulties encountered by previous installations.

It is our hope that the book will also stimulate new developments in this most dynamic and vital field of modern
technology.

George A. Bekey
Morton D. Schwartz
Los Angeles, California
September, 1971

Contributors to This Volume

JOHN C. BALL, Department of Psychiatry, Temple University, Philadelphia, Pennsylvania

MARION J. BALL, Department of Medical Physics, Temple University, Philadelphia, Pennsylvania

GEORGE A. BEKEY, Departments of Biomedical and Electrical Engineering, University of Southern California, Los Angeles, California

E. JACK BOND, McDonnell Automation Co., St. Louis, Missouri

LEE D. CADY, JR., The Center for the Critically Ill, Hollywood Presbyterian Hospital and Shock Research Unit, University of Southern California, Los Angeles, California

HOWARD CARRINGTON, The Center for the Critically Ill, Hollywood Presbyterian Hospital and Shock Research Unit, University of Southern California, Los Angeles, California

MORRIS F. COLLEN, Medical Methods Research, Permanente Medical Group, Oakland, California

E.C. DE LAND, Computer System Department, The RAND Corporation, Santa Monica, California

EUGENE A. MAGNIER, Computer Center, Temple University, Philadelphia, Pennsylvania

ROBERT F. MARONDE, Departments of Medicine and Pharmacology, University of Southern California School of Medicine, Los Angeles, California

ROY MARTIN, The Center for the Critically Ill, Hollywood Presbyterian Hospital and Shock Research Unit, University of Southern California, Los Angeles, California

MORTON D. SCHWARTZ, Department of Electrical Engineering (Biomedical), California State College, Long Beach, California

STANLEY SEIBERT, Pharmacy Services, L.A. County-USC
    Medical Center, Los Angeles, California

HERBERT SHUBIN, The Center for the Critically Ill,
    Hollywood Presbyterian Hospital and Shock Research
    Unit, University of Southern California, Los Angeles,
    California

GENE E. THOMPSON, Hospital Information Systems,
    Department of Hospitals, County of Los Angeles,
    Los Angeles, California

HOMER R. WARNER, Department of Biophysics and
    Bioengineering, University of Utah and Latter Day
    Saints Hospital, Salt Lake City, Utah

B.D. WAXMAN, National Center for Health Sciences Research
    and Development, Department of Health, Education
    and Welfare, Washington, D.C.

MAX H. WEIL, The Center for the Critically Ill,
    Hollywood Presbyterian Hospital and Shock Research
    Unit, University of Southern California, Los Angeles,
    California

Contents

1

Review of Hospital Information Systems *

E. C. DeLand and B. D. Waxman

Computer System Department
The RAND Corporation
Santa Monica, California
and
National Center for Health Sciences Research and Development
Department of Health, Education, and Welfare
Washington, D. C.

I. INTRODUCTION

A modern metropolitan hospital, perhaps more than any other social institution, is dependent on rapid and accurate information flow. Because, in the practice of modern medicine, correct information at the right time can be vital to save a life or prevent a catastrophe, the hospital is increasingly vulnerable to failures in the information net. Yet, relatively little has been done to modernize medical information-handling procedures. Although the amount of information is burgeoning in parallel with medical science

---

*
Reprinted from Handbook of Biomedical Information Systems (Encyclopedia Brittanica, Inc., Chicago, 1971), by permission of the publishers.

research, interest in reliable, automated medical information processing has only recently begun to grow.

Evolving social institutions relating to the delivery of medical care, urbanization of medical services, and increasing population have made medical data management a critical problem. Historically, organized medical information systems have been based upon manual methods of recording and transport. They have been adequate although incomplete, costly, burdensome, and slow. It has been generally estimated that, in an average hospital, the cost of patient record keeping and information handling is on the order of $20 per patient-day. The national magnitude of this cost, using the National Center for Health Statistics' estimate of 500 million hospital patient-days annually, is $10 billion [1]. Even if we presume 100% error, the daily cost is $10, and the national cost still $5 billion. This leads us to consider whether use of computer-based automation to support, supplement, or replace the all-manual methods would not (1) reduce the cost per patient-day and, simultaneously, (2) improve patient management through more timely, complete, and accurate information.

Proponents of automated methods argue the swiftness, timeliness, lack of duplication, and availability of the record, as well as more sophisticated benefits such as automatic statistical and analytical transformations of the data, and access to comparison cases and reference material by the ward-level physician. Skeptics argue the high cost of the initial system, retraining of personnel, lack of demonstrable benefit, inadequacy of current systems, and such subtle points as lack of record privacy and legality. Although the outcome

of this issue is not yet clear, it seems likely that we are now
in a transition period. Reduction of computer costs, development of software systems, and invention of facile interface
hardware will lead to highly organized, adequately cost-effec-
tive computer-based hospital information systems (HIS).

This paper reviews the current status in this country
of automated HIS, with particular emphasis on the involvement
of the U.S. Public Health Service (Department of Health,
Education, and Welfare) in the development and deployment of
these systems. Systems are being designed or developed
elsewhere in the world (particularly in Scandinavia, England,
and Japan), but we focus our attention on U.S. efforts.

The Public Health Service is immediately concerned
with potential technological aids because of its responsibility
to improve the delivery of health-care services. A growing
technology should have a profound effect on the service's
future plans. Properly developed and introduced, automated
systems could allow additional freedom and imagination for
policy decisions. Improperly introduced into the health-care
community, they could be quite costly and have negligible or
even adverse effects on policy.

In preparing this paper, it was necessary to clarify
the broad concept of HIS, and then describe subcategories in
more detail. We briefly describe these subcategories and
also attempt to summarize the degree of federal involvement.
However, a caveat is in order. It is obvious to even the most
casual observer that this new field is chaotic. Developments
are not yet coordinated via the literature and a total overview

is difficult to obtain. Even the federal government does not
have well-organized information systems, nor does it have an
information center for such activities. In consequence, any
effort to summarize the field will necessarily be incomplete.
This paper gathered available data in the Public Health Service
and from a search of the current literature. In addition, we
have looked briefly at industrial experience.

The category of HIS is quite broad; it includes all
potentially automated information sources, data transformation
and management requirements, and user information needs in
a patient-management facility. These requirements originate
in the several organizational elements of a medical center that
include the following.

     (1) The medical staff,

     (2) The admitting procedure,

     (3) Medical record keeping,

     (4) The nursing units,

     (5) Diagnostic services (x-ray, etc.),

     (6) Treatment services (radiology, etc.),

     (7) Hospital business and administration,

     (8) Hospital service operations (pharmacy, etc.), and

     (9) Communications (reception, etc.).

Each of these elements originates and uses patient information
[2]. Since patient information constitutes the kernel of the
general problem of patient management, improvements in
patient management should result from having more information more immediately available.

II. TECHNOLOGICAL CONSIDERATIONS

Technological developments applicable to the medical information problem have come, for the most part, from prior development and application in industry and the military. Computers are the primary tools for information systems, but, except for minor trends in research and patient monitoring, the computers in use are essentially identical to those used in nonmedical applications. However, very recently the pressing realization that medical systems are unique and complex has led to the evolution of specialized instruments and systems.

We must distinguish between the hardware and software of the information system; for medical application both will require considerable attention. The central hardware, a computer with a time-sharing system, is becoming fairly standard. However, the various peripheral terminals suitable for the numerous subenvironments of a medical institution are yet to be defined, despite several experiments (discussed below). Requirements at a nursing station differ from those at the admitting station or a clinical chemistry laboratory. If cost is not a major consideration, computer technology is equal to the task. In principle, when the several requirements are well known remote terminals will be available. Cost, however, is a consideration, and therefore remote terminals are usually designed with less power than they need to do the job. In the future one may reasonably expect terminal cost to continue to decrease and power to increase.

As for the software requirements, unfortunately, an applications program developed at one institution will generally not immediately be appropriate for another. However, the essential idea of a demonstrably useful program can be transferred, and the program either modified or rewritten. In this respect, software systems are similar to any other discipline, principles stand and libraries accumulate. In time, the operational essentials will be well known.

Nevertheless, medical system software must be evaluated on a deeper level. Several abortive designs have shown that a computer-system configuration may function perfectly for an information task and yet be useless in the medical environment. Usually, this is because the special applications programs required for that environment have not yet become cost effective or desirable for the problems and users at hand.

Because medically oriented tasks are considerably more complex than was at first realized, users have become disillusioned with the magic promise of computer systems. The applications programs for medical data management, to say nothing of more sophisticated programs such as hypothesis testing and patient management, do require considerably more subtlety than those for, say, industrial inventory control. For example, a rather arbitrary distinction may be drawn between a system for handling patient data and one for generating patient information. The former gathers and distributes the raw result of assaying or measuring patient parameters and variables. The latter is a consequence of raw-data transformation and analysis by either human or automatic means, and may involve judgmental data, or, say, statistical inference or modeling techniques. Presumably, information is considerably more useful than raw data because of its transformation, or its context, or perhaps, because of the exercise of rational inference. Automatic handling of patient data would certainly improve the efficiency and accuracy of data management, but an information system has the potential of contributing importantly to patient management. Although much, if not all, of the basic functional specifications for a hospital system may now be written, at this deeper level of patient-oriented programs much research is still required.

The broad system for computer-based medical information management in a health-care facility should properly be directed to the tasks of patient management, and therefore serve directly in the problems of patient-care administration, diagnosis, prognosis, and therapy. However, it is clear that there are problems of collecting, storing, transforming, and displaying the basic data on command. Consequently, efforts to design and implement data-management systems have most frequently been specific task-oriented projects in which the data, as well as the task, have some chance of definition. Such specific information systems are, for example, directed to the following services.

    (1) Nursing station
    (2) Admitting office
    (3) Business office
    (4) Historical medical records
    (5) Automated service

     (a) Clinical chemistry
     (b) Pharmacy
     (c) Dietary service
     (d) Blood bank
     (e) Radiology
     (f) Operating rooms
     (g) Other

(6) Current patient records

(7) Outpatient records

(8) Epidemiology

(9) Chronic disease records

(10) Research functions

(11) Automated history

(12) Continuing education

(13) Patient management

     (a) Diagnosis
     (b) Optimum therapy
     (c) Planning

(14) Statistical services

(15) Consulting services

     (a) Emergency
     (b) Information
     (c) Library
     (d) Referral

(16) Patient monitoring

(17) Emergency services

(18) Program planning and budgeting

(19) Community integration

Each of these services requires the development of the capacity to gather, manage, and display the data peculiar to that service – data as diverse as the services themselves. Thus, an automated hospital would not have an information

system, but a conglomeration of relatively discrete information subsystems. Presumably, these would then be integrated
into a smooth, centralized, information-handling capability
able to correlate and collate as much information from each
subsystem as necessary to provide a comprehensive medical
and/or administrative picture.

III. A TOTAL HOSPITAL INFORMATION SYSTEM

A total hospital information system is a computer-
based communication system capable of providing requisite
data management for every major medical and administrative
service in the hospital. At minimum, it must be able to gather,
store, and retrieve data pertinent to that service, retrieve and
display pertinent data gathered at other services, and perhaps
communicate with specialized data banks elsewhere (for
example, with the veteran's service or with Medicare). However, a truly successful and useful HIS must do much more
with the data: conversion, transformation, statistical analysis,
normalization, at least rudimentary model building and hypothesis testing (rules-of-thumb, etc.), and comparison with or
retrieval of reference material from the historical medical
records or the reference library (for example, the poison files
or tables, graphs, or rules for acid-base and fluid therapy).
Ideally, such a system should be able to support much more
complex procedures in patient management, for example,
automatic construction of simulations of the patient state for
trial therapy, support of physician decision using statistical
decision trees, and patient monitoring and screening. However,
these latter procedures are beyond the scope of this chapter.

Primarily, a HIS will contain the patient record, and must therefore acquire, organize, and retrieve these data on command. Current records are probably best kept in high-speed memory banks in the central computer so that they can be recalled or updated from remote terminals within a reasonably short time [3]. The main computer would also contain particular programs relating to particular activities at the remote terminals. Specialized terminals would be distinguished not only by the hardware appropriate to the local function, but also by the programs accessed to process data. For example, the business-office terminals are likely to continue to be small, peripheral computers that acquire current patient data from the central computer, update business records, predict room occupancy from nursing-unit terminals, maintain inventory from the pharmacy, and perform billing operations [4].

The admitting-office terminal, using current technology, would be an interactive device with which the patient converses. It would enter the interview data, order tests, and schedule and make room assignments. After the patient has answered a thorough and self-checking list of questions for the initial medical record, an initial problem list, determined tentatively by a computer, could be provided for the physician [5].

The nursing-station terminal is considerably more complicated, to accommodate the several activities there. It is likely to be an interactive console incorporating a CRT display and having various input devices. The nurse or clerk enters current information either by typewriter, multiple-choice answers using a form of stylus, or by monitoring devices and automatic transcription. Several terminals designed for aspects of this job have been demonstrated experimentally [6]. These terminals must also communicate physician orders to the pharmacy, laboratory, business office, or similar service. More research is needed on such problems as facile acquisition of nurses' and doctors' notes and complete physician summary, sufficiently flexible display, and, in general, those problems directly related to the man-machine interface.

The automated chemistry laboratory currently only punches cards or writes tapes that are then carried to the computer [7], but it is not a great step to insert the data automatically into the patient record for recall at the nursing station. The automation design for each laboratory service will naturally be different. Entry of pictorial data (x-ray, etc.) is as yet an unsolved problem, whereas the pharmacy orders and inventory control can be worked out in a variety of ways. A feasible automation of the pharmacy has been achieved at the Los Angeles County-University of Southern California Medical Center [8] (see Chapter 3).

Epidemiology, statistical services, research, and program-planning terminals now exist in a variety of forms, but for the most part these services currently use "batch" processing. The near future will bring "interactive" terminals whereby a user may share the computer with others via a remote terminal, scanning and analyzing banks of data essentially in a conversational mode with the computer. More sophisticated problems include interactive terminals used in support of physician decisions, as diagnostic and therapeutic aids, in clinical patient management, or for continuing or undergraduate education. All these uses seem possible in principle, but are quite difficult in actuality.

Despite these possibilities for the future, we must repeat the caveat that although feasibility may have been demonstrated in a variety of cases, these are generally far from a working, acceptable total system. The systems are already very useful in some cases, such as outpatient scheduling, automated pharmacy, clinical chemistry, and a few others; in most instances, however, research and development is still required to make such systems cost effective and useful in the medical environment. Nowhere does a complete system exist, but pieces certainly do, and reasonable predictions may be made so long as we are careful not to impose a strict time deadline.

IV. BACKGROUND AND DATA SUMMARY

Our objectives in this chapter were to (1) give a broad view of the components of an automated HIS, (2) briefly evaluate the cost and utility of current systems, and (3) estimate their future importance.

In collecting data, it became evident that there would be classification problems. First, the numerous ramifications of a HIS program and the interest of many federal agencies in similar or related systems made it inefficient if not inappropriate to attempt a government-wide catalogue of funded projects. Information was cross checked on several lists, such as the Research Grants Index and a number of grants

lists prepared by the respective granting agencies [9-24]. A
second problem, involving arbitrary decisions, was to determine which projects were truly relevant. Obviously, computer-
based research projects such as a statistical diagnostic program
are relevant, but not directly, and we chose to refer only to
those projects concerned with communication or information
gathering and data management within the hospital. Frequently,
too, actual information detailing each project is ambiguous.
For example, the information supplied may give categories in
which the investigators aspired to do research as well as
categories in which they actually engaged in research. Again,
if the researcher is working in several areas simultaneously,
it is difficult to determine the priorities he has placed on these
several areas. There is, therefore, an uncertainty in conclusions drawn about funds expended or areas emphasized.

A complete report is not currently available from the
Department of Defense relative to funds expended by that
department for HIS research and development. There are
several projects, but rather than conjecture, these data sources
are not included in this paper. The Army, Navy, and Air
Force all have significant programs in this area; but their
expenditures are considerably less than in the Department of
Health, Education and Welfare. However, the Veterans Administration has devoted approximately $6 million to the
development of a total HIS, and considerable work is currently
underway. Of course, the Veterans Administration hospitals
would greatly benefit by an automated network of information
systems [25-27].

Two significant nonfederal sources of research and
development funds for HIS must also be noted. The first is

speculative private industry; TRW, MITRE, North American, Aerospace, and others have developed certain aspects of information systems, some of which are directed particularly to the medical environment. The Systems Development Corporation, Bolt Beranek and Newman, Lockheed Corporation, and National Data Communications Corporation, among others, also have programs devoted to the development of a total HIS. This is a reasonably heavy commitment, but the total expenditure is unknown.

For private industry this field appears to be potentially quite lucrative. Unfortunately, it is not possible to directly transfer technical knowledge and developments available from industrial or military application, and the process of adaptation to the medical environment is exceptionally difficult for a variety of reasons. Development appears to be quite expensive in time and equipment. A reasonable estimate to bring up a minimally functioning total HIS is currently 200 experienced man-years. This figure will, of course, vary considerably; in particular, it will go down as nonfragile, applicable hardware and software subsystems are developed and become available in the literature and program libraries.

The second important nonfederal source is self-sponsored work in patient-care institutions. Total expenditures related to computers can be estimated from the number of computer installations in hospitals. Questionnaires were mailed to 2431 hospitals [28]. Of the 1251 responders, 543 used computers in some form, primarily in business applications. Assuming that the sample is representative, and extrapolating, we can infer that at least 1500 of the 2431 used computers. Of the 708 responding nonusers, 129 planned to install computers within 12 months. Based on the data of the questionnaire, it may be estimated that private sources furnish a considerable amount of computer funds. The fraction devoted to research and development cannot be estimated from available data but must be small, say, less than 10%. This rough estimate of hospital computer usage can furnish planning information regarding the potential market, even if it cannot be interpreted in terms of present R&D support.

V. SUBCATEGORIES OF HIS[*]

In searching the federal grants and contracts for data accumulation and analysis, it became apparent that actual current research and development is being done in six major categories of HIS.

(1) Medical records,

(2) Business-office transactions,

(3) Logistics,

(4) Diagnostic laboratory services,

(5) Physiological monitoring, and

(6) Total hospital information systems.

A. Medical Records

Subsumed under this category are three major activities important in the development of HIS: medical record

---

[*] Sources of data for the following summaries are from Public Health Service agencies only.

keeping; filing and retrieving orders, notes, and observations
of the medical staff; and the rudimentary library reference
function.

The medical record, normal commentary of the staff,
and related data are the central objects of the data-management
system (aside from the accounting and business-office functions).
In principle, it would seem relatively straightforward to record
and recall these data; in practice, the process is considerably
more exacting. The system must store and retrieve formalized
as well as textual information streams, numerical as well as
pictorial or analog data. The sheer volume of material is, on
the average, very high per patient since reports from several
services, the complete history, and daily charts and summaries
are in the record. Also, the input interface must be smooth
and direct. For example, should the physician entering reports
and orders deal directly with the computer interface or dictate
for entry by a clerk? And how does he verify that his orders
are correctly transcribed? Converse problems apply upon
retrieval and display of the data. Finally, there are problems
of encoding, of allowable vocabulary and nomenclature, of
efficient file structures, of statistical analysis, privacy, and
cost, to say nothing of the unique culture of the medical
community into which the technology must smoothly intrude.
Nonetheless, these tasks are tractable and adequate systems
will develop. Since 1962 the PHS has obligated approximately
$4.5 million for such development [29-32].

B. Business-Office Transactions

Included in this category are such activities as payroll,
billing procedures, accounting, and personnel operations.

These procedures are generally the simplest for the hospital to accomplish, primarily because such transactions are similar to other computer-programmed systems and constitute standard operating procedures. Hospitals usually automate this category first. About three times as many hospitals report using a computer for business-office transactions than for any other use.

There is only one government-funded project that could fairly be listed under this category; it is a demonstration of a shared hospital data system [33]. In this application, a time-sharing system was demonstrated in which 10 hospitals shared a computer for business-office data processing. One could say, however, that an "all or none" situation is operating in selecting from government-funded projects for this category. That is, all qualify because of an expected spin-off to patient care. On the other hand, none qualify because the major purposes for which the project was funded were in all instances representative of a patient-care management function. In sum, perhaps $2 million has been spent by the PHS in the development of business-office records.

C. Logistics

Under this category are the several departmental inventory control and distribution systems. These include, among others, the pharmacy, dietary, central supply, and the laundry services. Again, inventory control and distribution of supplies and equipment are computer functions well worked out by industry, although the medical environment imposes special requirements. A combination of industrial engineering

and systems analysis techniques are usually used to develop
an optimal system.

To date, the majority of hospitals simply maintain
depots on the nursing unit for each of these departmental
supplies. Freisen [34] has been developing a decentralized
concept for distributing supplies to the nursing unit, removing
the centralized depot on the unit, and establishing an area in
the patient room to store equipment for use. Also, the Freisen
concept centralizes the storage area for all equipment and
supplies for the hospital in a large receiving, storage, and
processing area so that distribution to the several rooms in
anticipation of demand requires careful and detailed planning

In addition to the inventory problem, the pharmacists
have also been concerned with automatic drug distribution
systems. An appropriate solution, unit doses individually
packaged and automatically dispensed, has been suggested,
but is difficult to implement. For instance, an appropriate
dispensing device for the nursing station, ward, or room,
needs to be developed that would be controlled by the central
information system. Problems in menu allocation and dietary
scheduling are also under study [35-38].

Finally, attempts are being made to develop efficient
schedules for outpatients, ambulatory clinic patients, patient
admission and interview, and bed utilization. Certain of these
queuing programs are in operation [39-41].

Approximately $4.25 million has been obligated in this
category by the PHS.

D. Diagnostic Laboratory

Under this category are included the clinical laboratory, radiology, and multiphasic screening. Their common central activity of furnishing diagnostic information also implies a data-handling function and a logistics function. The total PHS involvement to date is about $5 million [42-52]. For the x-ray department the computer may, in the future, provide assistance in reading the x-rays data. Currently, however, its functions are preparing the reports, scheduling, and automating the treatment protocol. Although these latter activities are fairly common, the former, automated image analysis, has proved to be a surprisingly refractory problem.

In multiphasic screening, the computer can assist in patient scheduling, monitoring some of the tests, data recording and analysis, initiating and supplementing patient records, and decision making. Collen [51] is representative of the PHS activity in this area where the current emphasis, in addition to developing the screening process itself, is in automation of data recording and analysis.

Automation of the clinical chemistry laboratories began with automatic analytic equipment. Subsequently, in a natural progression, results were automatically punched in computer-readable format, and finally read directly into a computer system where results may be transmitted to the ward. Demonstrations of feasibility for such data acquisition, transmission, and retrieval have considerably changed the complexion of future chemical laboratories even though the automatic equipment has by no means reached a state of final development. Refinement of the equipment and procedures will continue, but already the ready source of analytic data has spurred research efforts and resulted in a better understanding of population statistics [53]. Efforts are now underway to automatically incorporate the patient data into rudimentary mathematical models of blood and whole body chemistry for studies in acid-base physiology.

E. Physiological Monitoring

Included in this category are programs for the development of coronary care units, intensive care or critical care units, and operating room and cardiac catheterization laboratories. There are at least four distinct functions of physiological monitoring to be considered: detecting, recording, automatic analysis, and display of certain physiological signals and patient information. Early developments in this field took the view that the system was to be an early-warning device to detect and call attention to anomalies or dangerous trends. A more current view is that the automated system should do much more; in particular, it should do sufficient analysis of monitored variables, and sufficient transformation for display, to support usefully subsequent physician decision and action. That is not to say that the system will indicate the next step in patient management, but that, depending upon the circumstances, it will display information on demand to answer pertinent patient-management questions, for example, to predict the consequences of trial therapy. In this sense, the

computer system could be a much more useful tool than merely
a monitoring device.

Such a system would also be used in education and
training. In the Regional Medical Programs (RMP) the
physiological monitoring emphasis appears to be primarily on
coronary-care training programs. The RMP lists about 57
such projects in their November 1968 Directory of Programs.
This number also includes studies for feasibility of remote
facilities and curriculum planning for coronary-care training
programs. Funds for these projects are allocated to the
region and are listed in two categories: (1) planning grants
and (2) operational grants, of which the latter support the
coronary-care training programs.

There are nine projects, Myocardial Infarction
Research Units (MIRU), being funded by the National Heart
Institute at an estimated expenditure of $9. 1 million, some of
which may include subprojects in physiological monitoring.
Excluding the funds for the Myocardial Infarction Research
Units and money spent by the Regional Medical Program on
planning and training activities, the total PHS expenditure for
this category is $6, 508, 161 [54-60].

F. Total Hospital Information System

Using the definition given in this paper, there are in
the United States several projects under this category. However, an operating total hospital information system does not
now exist. Projects discussed in this category are dedicated
to developing such a system; some of them have operating

subsystems, while others do not. Other agencies of the
federal government (for example, the Air Force at Brooks
Air Force Base [26], and the Veterans Administration in
Washington [25]) support similar programs. The projects
discussed below are PHS programs.

A project entitled Data Automation Research and
Experimentation* proposed an investigation, through analytical and experimental means, of methods for recording and
communicating information in a modern, short-term, general
hospital. The focus was on the body of information relating
to an individual patient. During the period the project was
supported by the PHS, both the systems analysis and the
design of the system were accomplished. Implementation and
operation of the system were discussed in the final report to
the PHS as a continuing goal of the hospital. According to the
final report, a Control Data Corporation 3300 system with an
optical scanner has been selected (and contracted for purchase)
by the hospital to implement the system designed.

The project Demonstration of a Hospital Data Management System+ proposes to establish and operate a hospital
data-management system. It also proposes to (1) demonstrate
the interaction between the doctor's orders and patient care,
(2) demonstrate the responses of the patient to those care
procedures, and (3) evaluate performance and cost usage of
institutional resources. This project is in its third year, a

---

* Raymond B. Lake, Jr., Assistant Administrator, Memorial
  Hospital of Long Beach, Long Beach, California.
+ William A. Spencer, Texas Institute for Rehabilitation and
  Research, Houston, Texas.

critical one during which testing and evaluation will occur.
This facility is a small, 54-bed hospital. It will use the Baylor
University Computer Facility that has an IBM 360/50 and will
include video character display terminals.

The purpose of the Hospital Computer Project[*] is to
(1) explore the information processing requirements of the
urban general hospital, and (2) define and develop a hospital
information system to meet these requirements. Certain
well-specified, well-defined, modular information processing
activities will be implemented on an operational, hospital-wide
basis on one computer system. The major objective will be
to gain experience in providing reliable, efficient, continuous
service under conditions of actual use. Further, another
large multiaccess computer system is planned that will be
used entirely for research and development, exploring modes
of interaction, terminal devices, and information processing
algorithms suited to a variety of situations. Among these are
the use of conversational interaction techniques for the input
and communication of physicians orders, the direct entry of
histories, physical examinations, progress notes, and diagnostic reports, and the inquiry and generation of reports and
specific information. This is a 1000-bed teaching hospital
planning to implement operations in a stepwise, modular
fashion — giving considerable attention to ascertaining education requirements, the problems of implementation, and the
relative cost/value effectiveness. The computers to be used
are the PDP-9 and IBM 360/50.

---

[*] G. Octo Barnett, Massachusetts General Hospital, Boston.

In Demonstration of a Shared Hospital Information
System,[*] the hospital group will demonstrate the use of a
centrally located, shared computer for handling data for a
scattered group of hospitals. The computer is used as both a
switching device and a data pool to solve such urgent problems
as mounting clerical work load, poor communication between
departments, and poor information responses of ancillary
departments. Ten hospitals, ranging in size from 65 to 700
beds, share one computer, an IBM 360/50 with programmed
keyboard terminals.

The system developing under Computer Techniques in
Patient Care[†] also uses a patient-centered approach. A
patient profile is developed and the doctor's order serves as
a basis for coordinating the hospital services communication
system. Eventually, it is planned to integrate the financial
and administrative systems that are being developed with the
automated patient-care system. An evaluation of these
systems and the cost will be compared to the manual system
of communication for hospital care. This system is in use in
a pilot 80-bed unit of the City of Memphis hospitals. An
IBM 360/40 with programmed keyboards is the computer
system in use here.

---

[*] Walter S. Huff, Jr., Sisters of Third Order of St. Francis,
Peoria, Illinois.

[†] Glenn H. Clark, University of Tennessee School of Medicine,
Memphis.

For Computer Facilitation of Psychiatric Inpatient Care,* the hospital concerned plans to develop a communication system that will serve as a prototype for state, city, and federal psychiatric hospitals inpatient care. The standardization of behavioral observations is being used as the basis for development of the medical record. An automated nursing note has been developed. Development of the basic algorithms for classification of patients, diagnosis, prognosis, and therapy continues. This hospital has 400 beds. The computer in use is an IBM 1440 with Bunker Ramo video terminals.

The purpose of Psychiatric Data Automation† was to develop a hospital information system based on the existing data-handling techniques of that hospital. A demonstration of the experimental record system paralleling the manual record system was carried out on the special experimental patient-care unit. The computer system used was an IBM 1440. This is a large state psychiatric hospital having around 4500 patients.

An eighth project funded by the government is the one at the Veterans Administration Hospital in Washington, D. C. (Pilot AHIS) [25]. The Veterans Administration has been a pioneer in this field, having begun at Wadsworth VA Hospital in California in the early 1960's. The project was transferred to Washington, D. C., in the fall of 1964. The objectives of

---

* Bernard C. Glueck, Jr., Institute of Living, Hartford, Connecticut.

† Robert E. Graetz, Camarillo State Hospital, Camarillo, California.

the Pilot AHIS are to design, develop, test, install, and
operate an experimental hospital information system.
Following experience with the initial system, they plan to
complete the detailed design of an integrated system. Eleven
subsystems are being developed; two of these, the admissions
and dispositions and radiology, are currently being tested and
evaluated on all nursing units.

Three projects considered more relevant to this cate-
gory than to the other five categories are Computer-Based
Medical Interviewing Project (Warner Slack, University of
Wisconsin), Development and Use of Automated Nurse Notes
(Rita F. Stein, Indiana University), and Hospital Information
Systems, Optical Input/Output (Recording, Raymon Garrett,
Tulane University, New Orleans).

In summary, the PHS has spent approximately $10
million in recent years in this category. The operating system
goal is evidently quite difficult, but, as was discussed earlier,
we are in a transition period. With improving hardware and
accumulating software, it appears inevitable that adequate
data systems can be developed at an acceptable price. These
systems will then form the basis for extention into the more
sophisticated uses of an information system.

Finally, we should mention the significant industrial
activity directed toward design of total HIS. Inevitably, there
will be omissions in this list, we list here only those which
come to our attention.

    (1) The Bolt, Beranek, and Newman system was
         developed in conjunction with Massachusetts
         General Hospital. Its extensions are continuing

both at BBN and at Massachusetts General Hospital where the project of Octo Barnett is currently progressing.

(2) The several systems developed by the Systems Development Corporation have been tested, among other places, in Puerto Rico and at Mayo Clinic, Rochester. An active group continues this development at SDC.

(3) The TRW Corporation has proposed an automated system in conjunction with the University Medical School, Toronto, and elsewhere. Details of this system are not immediately available.

(4) Lockheed (now Technicon) has developed an extensive system and has several field tests and installations in operation. In addition, Lockheed contracted with the PHS to, briefly, analyze and report on the hospital information system problem. Among other results in this report, the information flow lines in a typical hospital were plotted and an algebra was developed to describe information flow quantitatively. A method was also designed to evaluate an arbitrary HIS [2].

(5) The IBM project with the Monmouth Medical Center, Monmouth, New Jersey, is representative of the many projects by IBM in both total HIS and in numerous subsystems for this application.

(6) A project at the Beaumont (Texas) Baptist Hospital is applying a system called REACH (Real-Time

Electronic Access Communications Corporation.
In this system, patient records, bed census, drug
files, medical records, business-office transactions, and other records and data are entered and
displayed on CRT consoles located through the
hospital. Most of the system is now operational
with a duplicated (small) central computer and 36
consoles in the first demonstration system.

(7) Arthur D. Little Corporation, the MITRE Corporation, The RAND Corporation, and others are also
involved at various levels in the development of
hospital information systems.

VI. CONCLUSIONS

We believe a number of conclusions can be gleaned
from the foregoing material.

Table I summarizes PHS expenditures for the several
HIS categories.

Although a considerably amount of money has been
spent on attempts to develop a total hospital information
system, the amount of money invested to date has not been
excessive in view of the complexity of the task.

At present, there is no fully functioning total hospital
information system and, with one or two exceptions, such
systems are not even employed on a piecemeal basis in the
delivery of medical care. To the extent that any success has
been achieved, it has been only in those instances where
institutions and/or investigators have implemented a relatively
limited set of objectives.

TABLE I

Total Grant and Contract Money Spent and Obligated for
Hospital Information System by the Public Health Service

Type of system	% of $32 million total grant
Diagnostic laboratory	15. 6
Physiologic monitoring	20. 5
Logistics	13. 3
Medical records	13. 3
Total HIS	31. 4
Other	5. 9

Although attempts to develop a total health information
system have been quite disappointing, there has nevertheless
been some rather remarkable success in at least two areas:
(1) the automation of the business functions of hospitals, and
(2) the automation of clinical chemistry laboratory procedures.

It seems noteworthy that so many hospitals throughout
the country have chosen to spend their own funds to install
computer systems to automate business procedures and, to a
somewhat lesser extent, clinical chemistry laboratories. It
is obvious that in both these instances large sums of money
have been spent without government subsidy; more than anything else this illustrates that in these two areas cost benefit
must have been recognized and achieved.

The discrepancy between the apparent success and
enthusiasm for the computer in the business office and laboratory as opposed to patient management suggests that in these
areas the need for the computer was more easily recognized.

There was a strong motivation to see these projects through to a successful operational stage. Thus, it may be that the lack of success in other areas has resulted from an inability of hospital administration to precisely define either the need for or usefulness of the computer in patient management. We would speculate that until other medical services, independent of external pressures, are capable of recognizing and demanding more efficient utilization of their time and services, attempts to automate these activities will continue to fail.

We recognize that the modern hospital is in fact not a single homogeneous activity, but rather a conglomeration of activities that, from a functional view, are only minimally related. It is reasonable, therefore, that the needs for increased efficiency as well as the recognition of these needs will develop at different rates. This differential awareness probably mitigates very heavily against the development of a total comprehensive hospital information system.

We believe that there are certain technological considerations that bear on the above observations. First, ignoring some of the organizational constraints to which we have alluded, it is quite possible that the failure of computer time sharing to develop on the schedules originally projected by our information scientists contributed in some way to the failures of many of the systems attempted. Quite simply, the technology was not equipped to provide simultaneously for the many divergent and data-rich requirements of the multitude of services that exist in any relatively large hospital. More importantly, however, is the possibility that what was technologically required was the development of a computer system

adaptable to an unevenly evolving need for computers among
the several services in the hospital, rather than to a total
frontal attack on all hospital services. The ultimate solution
to the hospital information problem may not be the development
of more useable time-sharing systems, but rather the development of a capability that can tie together discrete information-
handling capabilities as they develop at their own speed within
the several hospital services. Therefore, we submit that at
least one possible solution to the organizational problem,
which seems to be the crux, is to find some way to bring many
discrete activities together as they occur at their own rate of
development. In this sense, the notion of networking computers, especially computers not immediately compatible with
one another, may have a great deal more potential for the
evolution of a hospital information system than an attempt to
solve the problem with one very large machine. This very
general suggestion obviously needs a great deal more study,
but we believe that it has the virtue of adapting itself to reality,
rather than trying to impose upon the hospital an organizational
structure completely out of phase with the way hospital functions
are traditionally performed. It can be argued that what is
needed is a total revolution in the organization of our hospitals,
but this is much less likely to be achieved in the near future
than a solution that adapts itself to the way things actually are.

It is our opinion that, although every opportunity should
be taken to explore and examine new ideas and opportunities
in an attempt to develop hospital information systems, a great
deal of caution must be exercised in sponsoring activities that
do not appear to have the minimum ingredients for success.

We do not believe that we have identified all of these by any means; but we feel that past efforts give us certain insights and experience that begin to suggest certain minimal conditions, as well as new and as yet untried technological directions.

ACKNOWLEDGMENTS

The authors would like to express their appreciation to Bertha E. Bryant, Joseph E. Hayes, Jr., and Allan Janney, of the Health Care Technology Division, NCHSRD, HSMHA, DHEW for their assistance in the preparation of this paper. Any views expressed in this paper are those of the authors. They should not be interpreted as reflecting the views of The RAND Corporation or the official opinion or policy of any of its governmental or private research sponsors.

REFERENCES

1. National Center for Health Statistics, Vital and Health Statistics [13], No. 5, 1965 (last year published).

2. Analysis of Information Needs of Nursing Stations, Lockheed Missiles and Space Company, Sunnyvale, California, PB 186246, May, 1969.

3. W. B. Slack, et al., "A Computer-based Medical History System," New England Medicine, 274, 194 (1966).

4. G. O. Barnett, "Computers in Patient Care," New England Medicine, 279, 1321 (1968) (with bibliography).

5. J. Grossman, G. O. Barnett, M. McGuire, R. Greenes, and D. Swedlow, Automated Collection of Patient Histories, Laboratory of Computer Science, Massachusetts General Hospital, September 1, 1968.

6. R. D. Garrett, A. Levine, and R. O'Neill, Visual Input/ Output Devices for Hospital Information System, Tulane Automation Project, Tulane University School of Medicine, June 1969.

7. A. Peacock, S. L. Bunting, D. Brewer, E. Cotlove, and G. Z. Williams, "Data Processing in Clinical Chemistry," Clinical Chemistry, 11, No. 5, 595 (1965).

8. R. F. Maronde, Digital Computer and Patient Care Pilot Study, University of Southern California, Los Angeles, California, Project HS 84, 1970.

9. U. S. Department of Health, Education, and Welfare, Research Grants Index, National Institutes of Health, Division of Research Grants, Bethesda, Maryland, 1961-1967.

10. U. S. Department of Health, Education, and Welfare, Public Health Service, Public Health Service Grants and Awards – Fiscal Year 1967 Funds: Part I – Research, National Institutes of Health, Division of Research Grants, Public Health Service Publication No. 1798, Part I, Government Printing Office, Washington, D. C., June 30, 1967.

11. U. S. Veterans Administration, General Description of the Veterans Administration Pilot Automated Hospital Information System (AHIS), Veterans Administration, Washington, D. C. (revised April 1969; typewritten).

12. Myocardial Infarction Branch, "Annual Report," Myocardial Infarction Branch of the Artificial Heart – Myocardial Infarction Program, National Heart Institute, Bethesda, Maryland, July 1, 1967 – June 30, 1968, prepared May 31, 1968 (typewritten).

13. U. S. Department of Health, Education, and Welfare, Current Nursing Research Grants Supported by the Division of Nursing, Public Health Service Publication No. 1762, Government Printing Office, Washington, D. C., January 1969.

14. U. S. Department of Health, Education, and Welfare, The Use of Computers in Hospitals, Public Health Service Contract No. PH 110-233, Government Printing Office, Washington, D. C., 1968.

15. A. H. Turner, Jr., and D. A. Schmidt (eds.), Computers in Medicine Bibliography, Department of Radiology and the Medical Center Library, University of Missouri, Columbia, August 1966.

16. H. M. Hochberg, et al., "Automated Medical Communications Project," Medical Systems Development Laboratory, Internal Communication, Health Care Technology Program, National Center for Health Services Research and Development, Health Services and Mental Health Administration, Arlington, Virginia, May 1, 1969.

17. U.S. Department of Health, Education, and Welfare, Director of Regional Medical Programs, Health Services and Mental Health Administration, Public Health Service, Government Printing Office, Washington, D.C., November 1, 1968.

18. U.S. Department of Health, Education, and Welfare, Selected References to Computer Assisted Studies in Biomedical Research, National Institutes of Health, Division of Research Grants, Bethesda, Maryland Annual supplements, 1961-1968.

19. U.S. Department of Health, Education, and Welfare, Projects Activated Under the Hospital and Medical Facilities Research and Demonstration Grant Program, Bureau of Health Services, Division of Hospital and Medical Facilities, Research and Demonstration Grants Branch, Silver Spring, Maryland, May 1968.

20. G. O. Barnett, Report to the Computer Research Study Section, Research Grants Review Branch, Division of Research Grants, National Institutes of Health on Computer Applications in Medical Communication and Information Retrieval Systems as Related to the Improvement of Patient Care and the Medical Record, Laboratory of Computer Science, Massachusetts General Hospital, Boston, 1966.

21. U.S. Department of Health, Education, and Welfare, Journal References on Hospital Automation, Public Health Service, Division of Hospital and Medical Facilities, Health Facilities Services Branch, Silver Spring, Maryland, February 1967.

22. D. F. Cromwell, Q. R. Brown, and R. A. Kurzenake, Selected References: Automation of the Health Care Fields, Health Services and Mental Health Administration, National Center for Health Services Research and Development, Health Care Technology Program, Automation Section, Arlington, Virginia, October 1, 1968.

23. L. G. Gay, Bibliography on Hospital Automation, 1965, 1966, 1967, American Association of Medical Record Librarians, Chicago, Illinois, August 1968.

24. A. B. Summerfield and Sally Empey, Computer-Based Information Systems for Medicine: A Survey and Brief Discussion of Current Projects, Systems Development Corporation, Santa Monica, California, February 10, 1965.

25. Communication from Director of Health Information Systems Research Staff, Administration of Research Services (13D5), Department of Medicine and Surgery, Veterans Administration, Washington, D. C.

26. W. S. Beck, Automation for the Hospital of Tomorrow, Aerospace Medical Division, Air Force Systems Command, Brooks Air Force Base, Texas.

27. Preliminary Study of Inter-Hospital Communication Interface – Phase I, National Bureau of Standards Report No. 10-084, Project No. 6506421, April 1969.

28. M. A. Wolfe, T. A. Mulholland, and A. Cacciapaglia, Action Plan for a Specialized Information Center and Management Information System on Hospital Automation, Report III, Survey Analysis, Herner & Co., Washington, D. C., July 1968.

29. R. K. Ausman, Experimental Medical Records System, Health Research, Inc., Buffalo, New York, Project: HS 108.

30. R. E. Robinson, III, Demonstration of the Integration of Active Medical Records, Bowman-Gray School of Medicine, Winston-Salem, North Carolina, Project: HS 93.

31. L. L. Weed, Automation of a Problem Oriented Medical Record, Cleveland Metropolitan General Hospital, Cleveland, Ohio, Project: HM 578.

32. J. E. Schenthal, A System for Computer Processing of Medical Records, Tulane University, New Orleans, Louisiana, Project: FR 0006.

33. Walter Huff, Jr., Demonstration of a Shared Hospital Information System, Third Order of St. Francis Hospitals, Peoria, Illinois, Project: HM 504.

34. New Conveyor System Moves All Supplies, Modern
    Hospital, February 1965, p. 93 (article discusses concept
    of G. A. Freisen).

35. W. M. Heller, A Proposed Intra-Hospital Drug Distribu-
    tion System, Arkansas Medical Center Hospital, Little
    Rock, Project: HM 323.

36. W. W. Testor, A Study of Patient Care Involving a Unit
    Dose System, University of Iowa, Iowa City, Project:
    HM 328.

37. P. F. Parker, Guidelines for Practical Hospital Unit
    Dose System, University of Kentucky Research Foundation,
    Project: HS 103.

38. J. L. Balintfy and J. W. Sweeney, Linear Programming
    in Menu Planning in Hospitals, Tulane University, New
    Orleans, Louisiana, Project: HM 216.

39. A. G. Jessiman, Real Time Computer Services for
    Ambulatory Clinics, Peter Bent Brigham Hospital,
    Boston, Massachusetts, Project: HS 89.

40. L. W. Cronkhite, Control of Operations by Scheduling
    Using Terminals, Children's Hospital Medical Center,
    Boston, Massachusetts, Project: HS 113.

41. Charles Lebo, Hospital Data System: Automated Retrieval
    for Improved Admissions and Utilization, Presbyterian
    Medical Center, San Francisco, California, Project:
    108-66-288.

42. H. W. Jones, Development of a Clinical Laboratory Data
    Acquisition System, Phase II, Virginia Mason Foundation
    of Medical Research, Seattle, Washington, Project:
    GMHM 15581.

43. George Brecher, Automated Data Processing for Clinical
    Chemistry, University of California, San Francisco,
    California, Project: GM 14905.

44. R. L. Habig, Improvement in Automated Clinical
    Chemistry, Duke University Medical Center, Durham,
    North Carolina, Project: CD 315.

45. B. G. Lamson, Data Processing in a Medical Center,
    University of California, Los Angeles, Project: HM 300.

46. D. A. B. Lindberg, Hospital Laboratory Data Transmission and Retrieval, University of Missouri, Columbia, Project: HM 374.

47. David Seligson, Study of Data Systems for Clinical Pathology, Yale University, New Haven, Connecticut, Project: HS 75.

48. A. E. Rappaport, Computers – Automation: Impact on Laboratory Management, Youngstown Hospital Association, Youngstown, Ohio, Project: HS 60.

49. Seymour Werthamer, Hospital Communication and Laboratory Data Handling, Methodist Hospital of Brooklyn, New York, Project: CD 236.

50. G. S. Lodwick, A Systems Model for an Operating Radiology Department, University of Missouri, Columbia, Project: HM 477.

51. M. F. Collen, Health Service Research Center, Kaiser Foundation Research Institute, California, Project: CH 437.

52. H. R. Chinefield, Feasibility for Automated Multitest Laboratory Program (Pediatric), Kaiser Foundation Research Institute, California, Project: 86-67-251.

53. D. A. B. Lindberg, "Collection, Evaluation and Transmission of Hospital Laboratory Data," Methods of Information Medicine, 6, No. 3, 107 (1967).

54. H. R. Warner, Computer Facilities for College of Medicine, Latter-Day Saints Hospital, Salt Lake City, Utah, Project: FR 00012.

55. M. H. Weil, Development of Automated Systems for Critical Care Units, University of Southern California, Los Angeles, Project: HM 533.

56. R. W. Stacy, A Computer Resource for Physiological Data Acquisition and Analysis, University of North Carolina, Chapel Hill, Project: GM 15900.

57. S. R. Powers, Jr., On-Line Computer Study of Therapy for Human Shock, Albany Medical College, New York, Project: GM 15426.

38 E. C. DELAND AND B. D. WAXMAN

58. Paul Kezdi, On-Line Monitoring System for Intensive Care, Cox Coronary Care Institute, Dayton, Ohio, Project: HS 128.

59. Daniel Howland, The Nurse-Monitor in a Patient Care System, Ohio State University, Project: NU 95.

60. J. M. Evans, Coronary Care Unit Patient Monitoring Research and Development, George Washington University Hospital, Washington, D.C., Project: 86-62-213.

2

Status of Hospital Information Systems*

Morton D. Schwartz

Associate Professor, Electrical Engineering
California State College
Long Beach, California

I.   INTRODUCTION

Medical services are now the fastest rising item on
the consumer index.   They have soared by nearly 8% in 1969,
while the consumer index rose only a little over 3%.   Hospital
costs have been rising at nearly 16% per year for the past few
years.   The cost of a hospital room averaged $68 a day in
1969.   By 1975 it will reach $100 a day.   The nation's total
health bill for 1969 is estimated at $50 to $60 billion, or
approximately 6% of the Gross National Product.   By 1975,
the bill will be well over $100 billion and 8% of the projected
GNP.   In 1969, the federal government alone spent approximately $16 billion on medical care.   The health-care industry
now employs more than 300, 000 doctors, 640, 000 nurses, and
2 million hospital workers.   By 1975, it will employ 1. 5

*
Reprinted by permission of Hospital Progress from article
entitled "Status of Hospital Information Systems, " June 1970
by Morton D. Schwartz.

million doctors and nurses and 4. 5 million hospital workers.
As the absolute and proportionate costs of medical care rise,
new hospital management techniques must be developed to
provide the highest standard of health care at the lowest
possible cost.

II. POTENTIAL OF NEW MANAGEMENT TECHNIQUES

Computer-based hospital information systems (HIS)[*]
can provide new hospital management techniques. More than
10% of the hospitals in the U. S. are currently using some form
of electronic data processing equipment. This percentage is
rapidly growing, and a definite trend has been established.
The use of HIS systems is also expanding rapidly. For
example, one HIS supplier plans to install fully operational
HIS systems in 47 hospitals within the next 18 months. Other
HIS suppliers are in the process of developing similar systems
and anticipate a large market for their products. This means
that a hospital which plans on "keeping up" with the advanced
state of the art and wishes to be noted for its excellence in
patient care and utilization of advanced technological equipment must plan on eventually using an HIS system.

In order to assess the impact of the new management
techniques afforded by HIS on the spiraling costs of health-
care delivery systems, a course entitled "Hospital Information
Systems: Techniques and Applications" was held in 1969 and
1970 at the University of Southern California. The results of
this course are summarized in the following discussion and

---

[*] The abbreviation HIS for hospital information system is
used throughout this article in a generic sense.

indicate trends for the utilization of HIS systems in automating
the information flow and generating management tools for the
hospital.

III. HIS SYSTEM BASICS

A HIS system is defined as a high-speed, computer-
controlled, multistation, authorized access information flow
network for the hospital. It has business-office and patient-
care subsystems, and its function is to speed and simplify
administrative and medical information handling. The HIS
system interfaces with the hospital staff through the use of
data terminals located at the nursing stations and at strategic
points in the departments and service areas. As a result,
administrative and medical personnel have instantaneous
access to the electronic data banks for entry or retrieval of
patient data.

The HIS system stores, retrieves, routes, sorts, and
verifies the information flow. It can be designed to provide
patient medical histories, current medical records, statistical
summaries, and legal records. It can schedule medical tests
and maintain inventory control of beds and supplies. It can
provide current status of meal orders and accounting/billing
records. The computer makes it possible to automate the
information flow in the hospital and can undertake many tasks.
A brief description of potential HIS system tasks can be found
in the appendix.

Data entries and retrievals of computer-stored forms
or records are made from data terminals, except for accounts-
payable records which are accumulated and then processed.

English language should be used in communicating information
to the HIS data terminal system by means of touch-entry
devices, in order to simplify the training of hospital personnel
who will use the system. Touch-entry devices include light
pens, keyboards, programable keyboards, and selection
buttons. Hospital personnel should identify themselves when
using data terminals to ensure that only authorized personnel
have access to the patient's file. Identification and access
authorization are accomplished by inserting ID cards or
sequences of coded numbers into the data terminal.

The most flexible data terminals consist of displays
with television screens – cathode ray tubes (CRT's). Information is retrieved by computer generation of data in bright
letters and numbers on the screen. The touch entry device
is used to select data and/or "action words" which appear on
the display screen. Hospital personnel can select specific
data and categories for display or can complete displayed
forms or documents. When "action words" are selected on
the screen, the action selected is performed. This action can
range from calling up additional data displays to printing out
hard copies of data, to dispatching a message generated on
the screen to some department or service area.

IV. BENEFITS OF HIS SYSTEMS

The objectives of an HIS system are improved medical
information handling and more effective utilization of hospital
personnel, equipment, and facilities. Examples of HIS
systems currently in operation that satisfy these objectives

are the Baptist Hospital in Beaumont, Texas, and the St. Francis Hospital in Peoria, Illinois. These HIS systems are currently collecting and evaluating operational data to ascertain the cost effectiveness of HIS systems.

Some of the potential benefits which may be identified when the operational data mentioned above becomes available are as follows:

(1) Reduction in average length of stay through improved interdepartmental communications and availability of up-to-date medical records.

(2) Reduction in clerical workload, which allows the professional staff to devote more time to patient contact and care.

(3) Provision of care-oriented, computer-generated patient reports which interrelate and correlate pertinent data, such as a cumulative clinical laboratory report. Such a report would present all laboratory results to date in a summary format for the doctor.

(4) Provision of hospital operations-oriented, computer-generated reports which indicate to administration and management the current operating statistics for the hospital. These statistics include information on accounting, budgeting, financial data, bed census and occu-pancy data, medical records, abstracting and coding, and various medicolegal documents.

V.   GROWTH OF HIS SYSTEMS

Most HIS systems currently under development will probably be directed toward both business-office and patient-care data processing.   The initial emphasis of some systems has been directed toward business-office and accounting applications, but current and projected developments indicate a plan to supply a complete range of business-office and patient-care applications.   Progress has been slow; some HIS systems have been under development for five years and are still not ready for full hospital implementation.   However, considerable progress has been made recently.   St. Francis Hospital, Miami, Florida is an example of a leased HIS system in operation.   By 1972, there will be at least six suppliers of leased HIS systems in the U. S.

The anticipated patient-day costs for leased HIS services will range from $2 to $8 for hospitals with more than 200 beds.   The leased rates for smaller hospitals will probably be prohibitively high for some time.   For $2 a patient-day, the hospital would obtain interdepartmental communications, billing, and records for those items and services ordered through the HIS system.   However, the data terminals would not provide touch-entry devices; precoded data entry cards would have to be used.   At the other end of the cost spectrum ($8 a patient-day), a full range of information handling services would be provided, and CRT data terminals with touch-entry devices would be provided, producing a considerable degree of flexibility.   The $2 and $8 per patient-day figures include costs for both inpatient and outpatient activities.

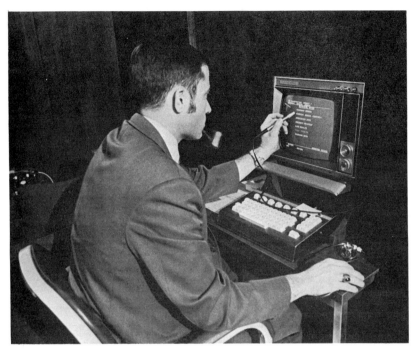

Fig. 1. A physician at El Camino Hospital, Mountain View, California uses the Technicon Medical Information System (MIS-I) to communicate his medical orders directly to the hospital's service departments. The system utilizes a network of video terminals like this, and accompanying silent high-speed printers at all nursing stations and ancillary departments.

VI. HIS SYSTEM REVIEW

HIS systems can be separated into four basic categories.

(1) <u>Comprehensive, multihospital HIS systems,</u> such as those at El Camino Hospital, Mountain View, California, (Figures 1 and 2) and St. Francis Hospital, Peoria, Illinois (Figures 3 to 8). These systems are large computer information systems. They have only recently been developed to

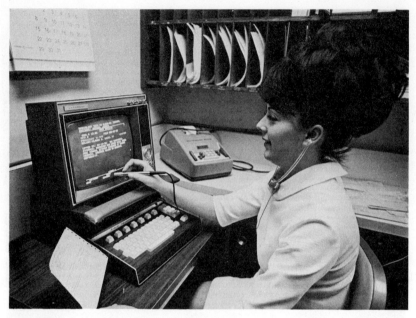

Fig. 2. A Radiology Technician at El Camino Hospital, Mountain View, California, listens to a radiologist's dictation of X-ray results which she enters into a video terminal for transmission to the patient's medical record.

provide data storage and retrieval capabilities and interdepartmental communications between admitting, business office, nursing stations, and medical services. They are designed to offer economies by time sharing their computer equipment among several hospitals. The potential advantages of time-shared systems are the sharing of hardware costs, software development costs, and common data banks for patient care and medical research.

(2) Comprehensive, single-hospital HIS systems, such as those at Los Angeles County-USC Medical Center, Los Angeles; St. Francis Hospital, Miami, Florida (see Figures

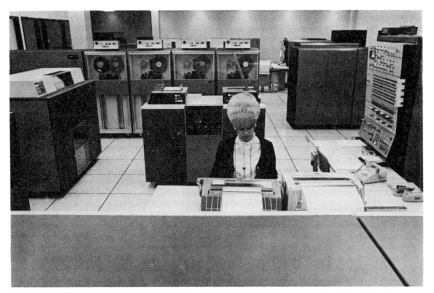

Fig. 3. Main computer complex of McDonnell Douglas Automation Company's hospital data processing service in Peoria, Illinois, has two identical large scale computers for processing both financial information and patient care information. Hospitals now using the Company's services transmit data to these computers over phone lines from terminals.

9 and 10); Kaiser Foundation Hospital, Oakland, California; St. John's Medical Center, Joplin, Missouri; and Baptist Hospital, Beaumont, Texas. These systems are similar to time-shared systems, except that they are used by a single hospital as a "dedicated system" rather than being shared by several hospitals.

(3) Business-office, multihospital HIS subsystems, such as those using the Minnesota Blue Cross Computer Center and those at Chester Hospital and Clinic, Dallas, Texas and Glenview Hospital, Fort Worth, Texas. These systems provide computerized office services to subscriber hospitals in the areas of patient billing, accounts receivable,

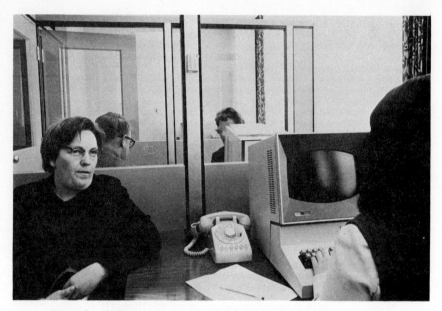

Fig. 4. Admitting room clerk takes information from patient on entering the hospital and advises all areas of the hospital of the patient's arrival through the computer system. (McDonnell Douglas Automation Co.)

general ledger, and payroll. Some time-shared computer centers supply a greater range of services than do others.

(4) Special-purpose, single-hospital HIS systems, such as those at Downstate Medical Center, New York City; Akron (Ohio) Children's Hospital; Texas Institute for Rehabilitation and Research, Houston; and Manchester (Connecticut) Memorial Hospital. These special-purpose systems will not be discussed any further in this review since they are not designed for general use.

The above categories comprise both business-office and patient-care subsystems of an HIS system. Examples of such subsystems are presented below.

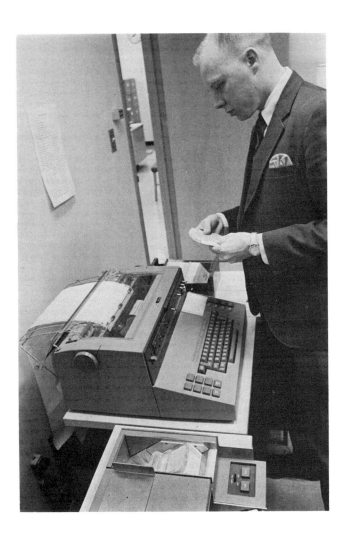

Fig. 5. Hospital attendant transmits accounting data to the computer through a terminal for processing. (McDonnell Douglas Automation Co.)

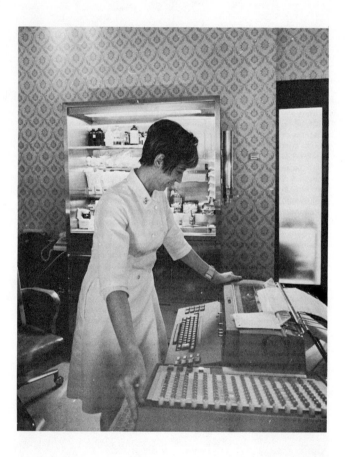

Fig. 6. Nurse in intensive care unit orders medications from the pharmacy for a patient by using the terminal. After processing her order, the computer system automatically prints a label, schedules the dosage and updates the drug inventory. (McDonnell Douglas Automation Co.)

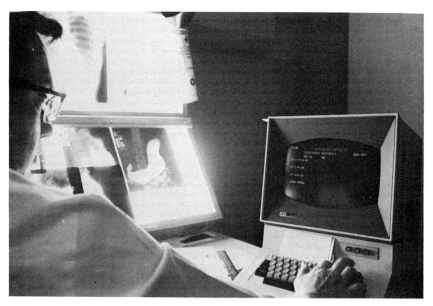

Fig. 7. Radiologist's diagnosis is entered on this terminal, and the narrative information appears on the screen before him. This information is transmitted both to the patient's
nursing station for use by the doctor and into the patient's
medical history file. (McDonnell Douglas Automation Co.)

VII. BUSINESS-OFFICE SUBSYSTEM

Business-office information is largely numeric and
concentrated geographically, and automated results can be
readily measured and compared with results of preexisting
techniques. Since business-office personnel are well
acquainted with quantitative methods and careful control,
business-office functions may be used as a starting point for
converting manual operations to HIS system operations.
Implementation of this subsystem will acquaint the hospital's
administration and part of its personnel with the advantages
and the constraints of electronic data processing. It offers

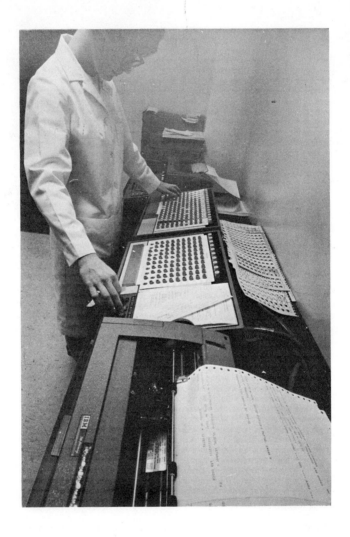

Fig. 8. The laboratory reports test results directly to the patient's nursing station and to the patient's file via a terminal. (McDonnell Douglas Automation Co.)

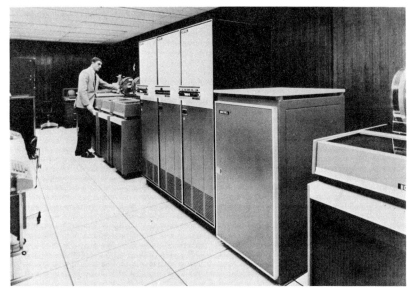

Fig. 9. Typical configuration of hospital communications control center for REACH System includes two modified Honeywell 516s, six disk drives, high speed line printer, two nine track tape drives, communications consoles, multi-line controller and CRT controller. The REACH System (Realtime Electronic Communications for Hospitals) is designed by National Data Communications, Inc.

an opportunity to train personnel in computer systems and has the potential to provide new management techniques in improved operations reporting and improved financial management. For these reasons, several suppliers have begun to develop business-office HIS subsystems.

An example of a business-office subsystem that has five basic areas of application is the one under evaluation at El Camino Hospital, Mountain View, California. This subsystem has been under development for 2-1/2 years and is

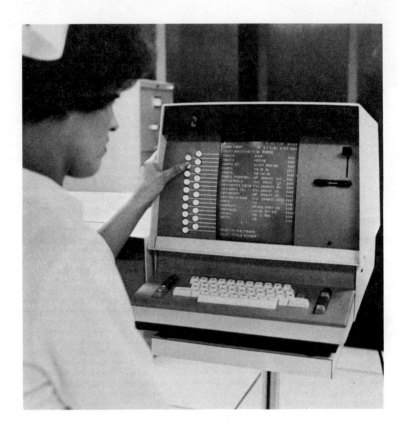

Fig. 10. Only instrument used by hospital personnel in
the operation of the REACH hospital communications system
is this duty station console manufactured to specification by
the Raytheon Company for National Data Communications,
Inc. Insertion of a specially coded badge, at right on console,
activates terminal. Doctors, nurses and other hospital
personnel perform their tasks through a series of selections
using the buttons aligned down left side of cathode ray tube.
Keyboard is used largely by skilled typists in admissions and
medical records.

now fully operational.   In addition to the business-office subsystem, El Camino Hospital is also in the process of evaluating a preliminary patient care subsystem on a limited number
of CRT data terminals.   The five business-office applications
are detailed in the following.

(1) Patient billing and accounts receivable.   The
patient billing/accounts receivable application provides a
patient accounting service in a batched* processing environment.   Transaction records in the form of keypunched cards
are prepared for each patient and for each charged item
accrued by that patient.   These transaction records may be
prepared from keypunch layout transmittal forms or from
source documents themselves.   They are generated by the
hospital and delivered to a central computer facility upon
conclusion of the hospital's working day or other daily cycle
cutoff time.   Included within these transactions are update
and/or correction cards to fixed tables in the computer
programs.   These tables contain such data as room/patient
type, physicians authorized/specialty   charge allocation/
charge descriptions, name, address, hospital number, and
billing cycle.   The tables are updated against each patient's
master record.   In addition to the patient's statement and
accounting breakdown of receivables, the subsystem also
generates both inpatient and outpatient Medicare billing forms.

---

*
Batch refers to "batch at a time processing." Several
computer programs can be batch processed at the same
time on one computer.

This application is designed to operate on a medium-size computer[*] with 64K core, tape drives, disk drives, and high speed printer. It is designed to interface with the general ledger program [application (4)] for allocation of charges to the proper chart of accounts summary and detail accumulations. The application will also interface with the HIS system under development in that data transactions will be accepted in a batch processing mode.

(2) Payroll application. This application provides a payroll service in a batch processing environment. Time cards in the form of keypunched cards or their equivalent are prepared for each employee. These cards are processed against the employee's master record, which contains the necessary data to extend gross pay and to compute deductions. The end result is the creation of payroll checks and various supporting documents, both of which enable the hospital to maintain effective control of the system. A few of the features that are included in this system are automatic accrual of employee benefits (i.e., sick, holiday, vacation); acceptance of prewritten checks (interim); eligibility checking for employee benefits; handling of pay rates different from employee's established rate; labor analysis reporting to the department that the employee actually worked; confidential payroll processing; and personnel statistical reporting by department of head counts and turnover rates. Besides the time cards, the hospital submits punched cards, using various

---

[*] This computer system is designed to be shared by many hospitals so that the total number of beds serviced can be about 3000.

transaction codes, to establish new employees on the master file, to set up or revise constant information on the employee (i. e. , rate, department assigned, address, deductions, etc.), and to show status changes. This application is designed to interface with the general ledger program [application (4)], passing to it the dollar values accumulated by the various liabilities and expense accounts.

(3) Accounts payable. This application provides an accounts-payable service in a batch data processing environment. A vendor name and address file is established, and the file controls the issuance of payment checks against valid due invoices. In addition to invoice register maintenance, the application interfaces with the general ledger in that input records are prepared as a result of accounts-payable activity for accumulation and posting to their associated general ledger accounts. The application can process interim payments to vendors which are written external to the check-writing program and incorporate these balances against the proper invoice register. The system also contains both internal and external balancing features and rejection and acceptance transaction listings.

(4) General ledger application. This application provides a general ledger service in a batch processing mode. Five types of transactions are entered into the general ledger system. They are: establish new accounts; update revenue budgets; update expense budgets; update allocation rates; and generate journal or adjusting entries. The hospital prepares journal and adjusting entries in the form of keypunched cards. These cards, along with computer-generated journal entries

from other business-office applications, are processed against
the general ledger master account records.   Trial balance
reports are created and once they are balanced, the hospital's
financial management reports are generated.   The management
report consist of the balance sheet, various income and
expense statements, and department cost-accounting reports.

(5) Inventory control application.   The inventory
control application provides an accounting technique for all
inventory items.   Direct issue items can be entered and displayed on an inventory status report and department supplies
expense report.

Provisions have been made for automatic inventory
price adjustments and backorder carry.   A purchasing action
report is keyed to a quarterly stores inventory catalog and
shows all items below minimum or above maximum, along
with last issue dates and total issues to date.

VIII.   PATIENT-CARE SUBSYSTEM

The Baptist Hospital in Beaumont, Texas, has installed
both business-office and patient-care subsystems at the same
time.   The functions of the business-office subsystem are
similar to those described above.   The patient-care subsystem
uses electronic equipment to store, process, and display the
patient-care information that a hospital needs in its daily
operation.   Computer program applications have been developed
for patient records, bed census list, drug files, employee
records, purchase order forms, patients' medical records,
and other hospital records.   The resulting information can be
displayed in printed form on any of the data terminals.   These

printed forms on the television screens are displayed in
sequence by pushing the appropriate touch entry devices.
Once the information is displayed on the screen, hospital
personnel can update records, order supplies, and perform
other routine functions by using lightpen devices or keys on
the data terminal keyboard to key in information.

In implementing the patient-care subsystem, all hospital personnel are assigned special identification entry codes
or badges that resemble a plastic card. If badges are used,
they are inserted into the badge reader to turn the television
screen on and to display a list of functions. These badges are
color and function coded according to the duties and responsibilities of the hospital personnel. When a badge is inserted
into the badge reader, the initial display corresponding to that
badge function is shown. The initial display lists those tasks
or functions for which a hospital department is responsible.
Thus, nurses' badges produce only a nurse's display, etc. No
person can display records for which he has no need or job
responsibility. Nurses can work only with nursing functions,
pharmacy can work only with pharmacy functions, etc. The
individual badges protect and guarantee the confidential nature
of all information within the HIS system.

The data terminals are located at duty stations throughout the hospital as required. Some duty stations, such as
dietary, may have only printers. The data terminal is the
only piece of equipment which hospital personnel use to enter
data when communicating with the HIS system. By inserting
the badge into the badge reader, the data terminal is automatically turned on, the badge holder is identified, and an initial

display is shown on the television screen. The initial display lists the tasks that can be done. Viewing records to see if they are complete, ordering a medication or a central supply item, and charting patient data are examples of the three main tasks that can be done. A task usually involves a sequence of screen displays.

To the side of the television screen is a light-pen device or selection buttons. The light pen is used, or the selection button is pushed, to select a particular task. The display will show all of the information that has been added to the many different hospital records. Information is entered into the HIS system by either selecting a series of words to form a message or using the keys on the keyboard to enter the information on the screens. The keyboard is similar to that of a standard typewriter. The information is displayed in capital letters as it is keyed in on the screen, and corrections or changes can be made before storing it in the system. The new information is immediately available for display at any of the data terminals throughout the hospital. After each task is completed, the initial display is shown again in case the person operating the equipment wishes to perform additional tasks. When a task is completed, the nurse, technician, or doctor uses the appropriate codes or pushes the badge release lever to remove the badge from the badge reader. The terminal is then automatically turned off.

The patient-care and business-office subsystems provide the hospital administrator with the following management tools and administrative control.

(1) An invoice cannot be paid more than once.

(2) Patient service charges cannot vary among patients, since all charges are obtained from a computer-based file approved by the administrator.

(3) A patient's account cannot be lost.

(4) Through the use of computer-based inventory control, inventories cannot reach undesirable high or low levels.

(5) Orders cannot be lost by service departments since the HIS system "reminds" personnel of any unfilled orders.

(6) Authorized signatures are obtained whenever entries or retrievals are made on the data terminal.

(7) Cash flow can be monitored on a current basis.

(8) Dollar value for each test and treatment can be obtained on a monthly basis.

IX. COST-BENEFIT TRADE OFFS

A hospital must be willing to increase its patient-day costs by $2 to $8 for a full HIS system and $0.50 to $1 for the business-office subsystem only. The resulting benefits may include reducing the length of patient stay, increasing bed occupancy, providing better management reports and tools, improving interdepartmental communications, reducing the possibility of transcription errors, and establishing a data bank for teaching and research purposes. An HIS system has the additional potential of uncovering lost or erroneous charges. This benefit alone could possibly constitute one of the major savings.

Most of these benefits will produce savings to offset the HIS system costs. However, no measure of cost effectiveness can be made at this time since the extent to which hospitals can employ HIS systems to take advantage of labor and material cost offsetting when changing from a manual to a HIS system has not been fully assessed at this time. However, considerable data obtained over many months of operation should be shortly available from the HIS systems at Baptist Hospital, Beaumont, Texas, and St. Francis Hospital, Peoria, Illinois. The resulting trade off of manual system costs against HIS system costs will, in the end, determine the resulting economics and cost effectiveness. The problem is further compounded by the many intangibles involved, such as the cost of computer-generated management reports for hospital administrators, which have no direct dollar return but are of benefit to the overall operation of the hospital.

X.   APPENDIX

This appendix[*] presents an overview of the potential HIS applications that are under consideration by various suppliers developing HIS systems. The objective in providing such a list is to indicate the direction which such efforts are taking.

Before the HIS tasks can be defined, a set of files must be established to store the data for entry or retrieval purposes.

---

[*] Summarizes, in part, a presentation made by Dr. William T. Blessum, director of the Medical Computer Facility, University of California at Irvine, to the Summer Course on Hospital Information Systems, University of Southern California, Los Angeles, July 1969.

The following set of files is extensive in scope and allows a comprehensive HIS system to be developed: ancillary services, accounting, inventory, pending, noncompleted, drug index, medical records, outpatient records, doctors' orders, reservations and bed-available, result collector, registry, blood donor registry, inpatient records (may contain patient charts), personnel, poison index, preadmission, and glossary of terms used in HIS system.

The above files are then used in the following HIS application areas to store data entries for later retrieval. Each HIS task is an application area which provides billing and accounting, laboratory data processing, registry and indexing, administrative controls, or patient-care reports.

A.   Business-Office Subsystem, Billing and Accounting

Hospital billing function. Contains a list of the accounting files of all charges applied to a patient's account and produces detailed bills at specific intervals, with a summary and prorated third-party bill on discharge.

Admission/discharge. Used for inpatient and outpatient admission and discharge and includes the following.

(1) Updating of reservations and bed-available files.

(2) Establishment of inpatient and outpatient records, both in abbreviated form and in a complete form.

(3) Medical records file, patient accounting file, and doctors' orders file.

Cost-accounting function. Provides for the analysis and accumulation of actual costs incurred. The supporting data is used for gained reimbursement from Medicare and for

adjusting charges in the following year to reflect actual costs.
The system produces reports at department levels for financial control and operating control.

Payroll function. Provides all payroll and associated
accounting transactions and services for hospital personnel.

Open accounts receivable. Provides inquiry capability
at detail level; updates bill at detail level; periodically updates
open accounts; transfers record to closed A/R on zero balance.

Purchasing function. Obtains products and services
needed in the hospital and updates department records to
reflect expenditures. It provides for two kinds of purchasing:
emergency orders and routine orders (to be accumulated by
the vendor and processed on a 24-hour basis). In addition,
it updates inventory files to reflect items on order and prices
and records the inventory file.

Accounts-payable function. Produces checks for
vendors, check register, and list by vendors of items purchased along with payment record. Updates departmental
financial records to show all activity on a daily basis, thereby
making it possible to generate real-time status reports of any
account. Input and output is on a batch and random basis for
status report of any account.

Outpatient accounting function. Provides accounts
receivable function for outpatients.

General ledger function. Produces general ledger
reports as follows.

(1) Detail level for departmental heads.

(2) Summary level for administration.

(3) Detail income report showing all actual income
for month and year-to-date figures.

(4) Detail expense report, similar to income report.

B. Patient-Care Subsystem, Laboratory Data Processing

EKG analysis. Automates collection, analysis, and
reporting of EKG results. EKG's can be processed in real-
time (monitoring or other high priority); in real-time accession with batch processing; or with automated or nonautomated
off-line accession and batch processing.

Laboratory analysis function. Provides computer-
assisted analysis of test results. (Was the test valid? Should
it be rescheduled? Did the test show a critical condition?)
Updates patient records showing results. Posts completion
in doctors' orders file and accounting files.

Service (labs) report function. Checks results of tests
when reported directly into "result collector" file, and produces reports from "result collector" file for the medical
record (by patient) at intervals, adjusting to system, terminal,
and ward-clerk/office-staff schedules. Prints or displays
report at nursing station when test is reported, and posts
entries to patient medical records and in billing accounting
file.

C. Patient-Care Subsystem, Registry and Indexing

Registry function. Maintains separate registry files
by medical subject such as psychiatric, retardation, alco-
holism, birth defects, crippled children and adults, tubercu-
losis, stroke, heart and tumor. These files contain basic

medical data, diagnosis, treatment record, and results of
treatment.

Blood donor registry. Maintains current files on
donors, including their location, types, and donating groups.
Lists of last year's donors are prepared for collection groups,
and notices of dates and times for each donating group are
produced and mailed to the participants.

Poison index. Maintains up-to-date poison control
index for random retrieval from hospital wards, emergency
rooms, physicians' offices, or poison control center. The
index lists poisons by their brand names, chemical names,
industrial usage types, and toxic effects. The file also contains currently recommended treatments.

Departmental indexing function. Provides the individual departments with a tool for collecting and cataloging data
that is pertinent to their particular interest. These indexes
can be used for diagnostic tools and quality control. Produces
updated monthly report showing one or more of the following
for new additions: alphabetical listing, hospital number listing,
diagnostic breakdown, departmental accession number listing,
and frequency distribution of diagnosis. The following indexes
are also available: surgical pathology, cytology, clinical
pathology, autopsy lab, radiology, EKG, and EEG.

Drug index. Maintains information concerning drugs,
indexed in a fashion similar to the Physician's Desk Reference.

D. Patient-Care Subsystem, Administrative Controls

Patient transfer. Updates patient record for transfer
from one bed location to another and possibly from one nursing

station to another. Pending doctors' orders must be reprinted
at the new nurses' station. When transfer occurs, the service
departments must be informed of the new bed location.

Service scheduling. Prints a list of work to be done in
each of the service departments for a shift of personnel.

Nursing scheduling. Prints or displays a list in the
chief nurse's office and the administration office of the names
and types of nurses required for each floor for each shift.
This schedule is developed by examining patient status, type
of service required, bed status, personnel files, and pending
doctors' orders.

Maintenance scheduling function. Provides printout
of routine plan maintenance procedures to be carried out by
in-house maintenance staff and outside vendors. Maintain
records of completed work, showing date completed, materials
used, man-hours needed, and actual costs. Makes it possible
to alter schedules when the need arises, when new procedures
are initiated, when current practices are inadequate, etc.

Schedules maintenance of in-house medical instruments,
such as recalibration of electronic metering devices, scales,
etc.

Dietary function. Provides daily printout of each
patient's menu, along with a list and summary report used
for meal production planning. Provides for individual menu
selection via the nursing station. The food usage and services
required are reported at the department level.

Terminology and procedures definition and inquiry
function. Develops and maintains a glossary of terms to be

used within the entire HIS system. Displays, upon request, the definition of any medical term or procedural term utilized in the system.

Inventory control function. Provides for control of consumable and nonconsumable items, either patient-care directed or non-patient-care directed. Provides accurate and timely reports on existing store items, including usage analysis reports which show the necessity of either increasing or deleting items. Provides both hospital-wide and departmental level reports that contribute to cost accounting and property control. Provides departmental reports showing estimated reordering times and quantities.

Census function. Provides clocked or demand inquiry printout of census by nursing station and type of service.

Bed availability function. Provides, on request, a list of available beds by service type.

E. Patient-Care Subsystem, Patient-Care Records

Nurses' notes function. Provides a means for incorporating nurses' notes and physicians' notes into the medical record file for the purpose of reporting patient condition to the physician and subsequent nursing shifts. The notes may be coded or in English form, as required, and are reported via remote terminal to the patient record.

Preadmission. Provides for collection of data from the patient and the physician concerning type of service, credit, insurance, medical data, basic vital statistics, and

preadmission physician orders. All this information is held
in a preadmission file, pending actual admission.

Physicians' orders function. Provides a means of
entering physicians' orders for patient care into the system.
The orders are verified and distributed to various active
ancillary services files, to the appropriate nurses' station,
to accounting files for billing purposes, and to inventory files
for posting. The orders are maintained in a "pending" file
and, if treatment or care is not completed, a separate entry
is made into a "not-completed" file for review by the medical
staff.

Orders for medications are checked against the drug
index file for dosage range, pharmacologic antagonism, and
contraindications. In addition, if special instructions for
administration or observation of side effects are necessary,
these are communicated to the nursing station and/or physicians' office.

The application ultimately includes PRN orders to be
carried out, only if specific criteria (e. g., a test result in a
certain range or a given change or lack of change in a patient's
condition) are met.

Medical records maintenance. Provides for the
manual and automated review of existing medical records for
the hospital and practitioner and also includes the following.

(1) Removal of records of deceased patients into
deactivated records file, six months to one year
after death.

(2) Scanning of records for incompleteness or lack of diagnosis.

(3) Routine file additions for result reporting and notes.

Outpatient result reporting. Provides for clinical and ancillary service reports, originated by physicians' orders, to be reported to the data management system and incorporated into the patient's medical record.

Case history and physical. This application area represents one of the most difficult and urgent of all application areas. Three basic alternatives exist with regard to entering case history and physical information.

(1) Entry of material in narrative form only.

(2) Entry of historical and physical data in narrative form, with diagnostic information entered in a coded or machine-readable form.

(3) Entry of all historical and physical information in coded or machine-readable form.

By means of central dictation systems doctors may narrate history and physical data into a central stenographic "pool." The "stenographers" will "type" the information directly into the computerized medical record in an on-line, real-time mode. Dictation technique will include verbal delimiters such as "chief complaints," "history of present illness," "past history," "family history," and similar categories for the physical examination data.

Physician display function. Provides the physician with direct access to his patients' medical records, including

hospital status; to his own records; and to various files in
the data management system. Access is achieved by remote
terminal on the nursing floor or at the physician's office in
a doctors' office building.

3

Electronic Data Processing
of Prescriptions *

Robert F. Maronde
Professor of Medicine and Pharmacology
University of Southern California School of Medicine
Los Angeles, California
and
Stanley Seibert
Director of Pharmacy Services
Los Angeles County - USC Medical Center
Los Angeles, California

I. INTRODUCTION

The Los Angeles County - University of Southern California
Medical Center is one of the largest in the world. Over
600, 000 outpatient prescriptions are processed yearly. These
prescriptions are being processed, as a part of the drug dispensing system, by means of computer terminals.

This chapter describes in general terms some of the major
aspects of the data processing system, including data entry,
user codes, and types of data which may be retrieved from the
system. A recently completed study of prescribing patterns
is used as an example of the usefulness of the computer system
in identifying possible problem areas within a major hospital.

---

* A portion of this chapter has been adapted from an article
    entitled "A Study of Prescribing Patterns," by R. F. Maronde,
    P. V. Lee, M. McCarron, and S. Seibert, published in
    Medical Care, 9, No. 5, and reproduced by permission of
    the publishers.

In this study, three types of undesirable or inappropriate prescriptions were defined and identified by physicians and pharmacists at the Medical Center. These are (1) excessive drug
quantities specified in individual prescriptions, (2) undesirably
frequent prescriptions for the same drug, and (3) inappropriate
concurrent prescriptions for different drugs. In addition, the
data processing system makes it possible to find numerous
examples of concurrent prescriptions of two different drug
products which could result in serious drug interaction or
potentiation.

II. COMPUTER TECHNIQUES

A. Input of Prescription Data

Entry of prescription drug data into the data processing
system may be performed on-line or off-line. Off-line data
entry is usually in one of two forms: punched cards or tape.
Punched cards, or variants such as mark-sense cards or
optical scan forms, may result in an unacceptable incidence
of error. Error checks and error corrections are relatively
inefficient, and filing and updating of the cards are time con-
suming and cumbersome. Because of these limitations, data
entry is usually carried out separately from the actual prescription processing. Most commonly the actual data acquisition is retrospective. Since data acquisition of this type is
not an integral part of the prescription processing, editing,
error checks, and updating of data files are carried out under
circumstances that make it difficult to assure the validity of
the data.

1. Off-Line Input

Off-line tape data entry is accomplished by an encoder
with a typewriter keyboard. Error checks are more easily
made with tape systems than with punched cards, in most

instances. However, error correction and label generation
are not as easily handled as with the existing system of
prescription processing. Therefore, prescription data acquisition using an encoder again would be carried out separately
from the prescription processing. The disadvantages cited
above under the discussion of data entry by use of punched
cards will also apply here.

2. On-Line Input

On-line data entry requires a terminal connected by
telephone line or cable to the central processing unit (CPU).
We have used three variants of remote terminals; typewriter
keyboard terminal, cathode ray terminal (CRT) with a typewriter keyboard, and a push-button terminal with a typewriter
keyboard. Remote terminals allow data to be entered in an
abbreviated form, expanded by the CPU, and printed and/or
displayed at the site of entry for error checks and for verification of data. After verification has been completed a small
printer at the terminal site can print a label for the drug
container, a prescription for the physician, or a printed entry
to affix to the patient's chart. We use CRT's with a typewriter
keyboard for prescription processing, including error checks
and verification (Figs. 1 and 2). This provides a rapid form
of prescription processing that has been well accepted by the
pharmacist [1,2].

3. User Codes

The drug item, dosage, and directions for taking the drug
item are entered in an abbreviated form that relates to the
drug name and to the content of the physician's instruction.
For example, L-10 is the abbreviation for chlordiazepoxide
10-mg capsules, and TIL3D is the abbreviation for "take one
capsule three times daily. " These are called user codes and
have the advantage of being much easier to relate to the actual

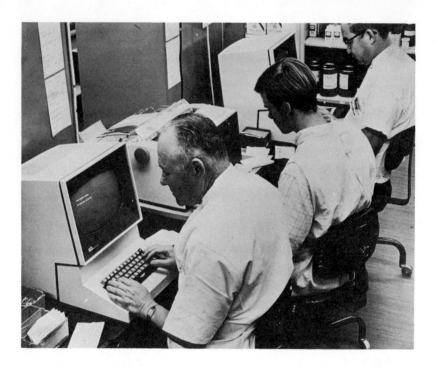

Fig. 1. Typical terminal for entry and verification of prescription data.

L.A.C./U.S.C. MEDICAL CENTER, 1200 N. STATE ST., L.A.
235-79-01   #71090-5001-0/2
Harrison,George
Take 1 Capsule 4 Times A Day
*TAKE ON EMPTY STOMACH-
DISCARD AFTER 1 YEAR-TAKE
WITHOUT MILK

100 Tetracycline 250mg,dd
Dr.Jones
IJK 03/31/71   1L COPD1

Keep Out of the Reach of Children

Fig. 2. Label for drug container as printed by terminal.

meaning than a series of numbers or letters that have little or
no discernible relationship to the actual content of the message. The development of user codes is an important facet of
medical data processing and deserves some comment. A variety of different sets of medical data show similar curves
when the occurrence of individual variables are plotted against
the total number of variables within the set. Twenty-eight
drug items out of a formulary of over 1400 items account for
50% of all prescriptions, and 166 drug items account for 90%
of all prescriptions; 15 diagnoses account for 50% of all diagnoses made, and 40 diagnoses account for 90% of all diagnoses
made, etc. This general curve applies to interpretations of
x rays, electrocardiographic diagnoses, laboratory results,
and many other types of medical data that one might want to
enter by computer terminal. The problem is to define accurately what actually comprises the high-frequency data and to
fuse terminology. Laennec's cirrhosis and alcoholic cirrhosis
may mean the same thing to a physician, but to a computer
they are not related unless a table of synonyms is referred to
by the programs for the computer. A user code provides a
standard terminology so that building tables of synonyms, usually a complex and laborious programming effort, can be
minimized. Furthermore, the entry of user codes is easier
than typing the complete message and does not tie up the computer for as long a time. The user code for the high-frequency data is readily learned by the user, particularly if he
has been involved in the development of the code in a collaboration with the EDP staff.

B. Storage of Prescription Data

The main types of EDP file storage of prescription data
that may be used are three in number. These are punched
card files, tape, and random access files such as disks or

data cells. Card files are bulky, subject to damage, and they
are comparatively difficult to store, maintain, and update.
Accessing card files for the purpose of data analysis is laborious. Because of this, card files are impractical for the generation of warnings related to contraindicated, concurrently
prescribed drugs or previous drug sensitivities at the time the
prescription is being processed. Tape files are faster to
search than cards but slower than disks or data cells because
accessing a tape requires a linear search. Tape files are
also too slow for high-volume prescription processing associated with analysis of a patient's drug file at the time the prescription is being processed. We therefore use disk files.
We process over 600, 000 prescriptions annually for a patient
population that exceeds 200, 000, and we can justify the application of a sophisticated EDP system because of this volume.

III.   REPORTS AND ANALYSES

The types of reports and analyses that are being carried
out have proven to be of value to the Los Angeles County-USC
Medical Center administration. A partial list of these is presented below.

A.   Printed Reports

Printed reports are used by the Therapeutic Committee,
pharmacist, Hospital Administrator, Medical Director, or
house staff.

(1)   Cost ranking of all prescriptions by drug item.

(2)   Frequency ranking of all prescriptions by drug item,
      as for example, in Table I.

(3)   Reports on all prescriptions for narcotic drugs that
      exceed a defined amount or defined frequency, as,
      for example, in the data of Table II.

Table 1. Summary of Pharmacy Activity for 2/01/70 to 2/28/70 Report Ranked by Frequency of Prescription

DRUG NAME	DRUG CODE	# OF RX	% OF TOT	CUM %	QTY	MEAN	COST	MEAN COST	% OF TOT
PROPOXYPHENE 65MG,LY	D65	4791	8.41	8.4	282085	58.9	$10493.14	$2.19	9.046
HYDROCHLOROTHIAZIDE 50MG,AB	E550	1754	3.08	11.5	233756	133.3	$2090.67	$1.23	1.802
CHLORDIAZEPOXIDE 10MG	L10	1702	2.99	14.5	168352	98.9	$5555.53	$3.26	4.789
ALUMINUM HYD GEL-MAGNESIUM HYDROXIDE	106	1647	2.89	17.4	17157	10.4	$1115.21	$.68	.961
POTASSIUM CHLORIDE 10% SYRUP,LAC	KS	1580	2.77	20.1	2121383	1342.6	$698.49	$.44	.602
MULTIVITAMIN TABLETS	156	1528	2.68	22.8	1955	1.3	$508.30	$.33	.438
DIAZEPAM 5MG	VL5	1454	2.55	25.4	126651	87.1	$4812.68	$3.31	4.149
ASPIRIN 300MG CODEINE 30MG,BW	ASAC3	1197	2.10	27.5	37388	31.2	$1005.65	$.84	.867
TETRACYCLINE 250MG,DD	TC250	904	1.59	29.1	42780	47.3	$834.19	$.92	.719
PHENOXYMETHYL PENICILLIN POTASSIUM 250MG,WY	PNVK	894	1.57	30.6	33942	38.0	$2033.04	$2.27	1.753
DIGOXIN 0.25MG,DR	DGX	843	1.48	32.1	83526	99.1	$183.63	$.22	.158
DIPHENYLHYDANTION 100MG,PD	DL100	740	1.30	33.4	153048	206.8	$442.04	$.60	.381
PHENOBARBITAL 30MG,ST	P830	699	1.23	34.6	105313	150.7	$52.53	$.08	.045
CHLORAL HYDRATE 500MG,FT	CH500	656	1.15	35.8	30056	45.8	$228.33	$.35	.197
CLINITEST TABLETS	128	653	1.15	36.9	1013	1.6	$1296.64	$1.99	1.118
CHLORPHENIRAMINE 4MG,KS	CT4	649	1.14	38.1	31839	49.1	$22.21	$.03	.019
GLYCERYL GUAIACOLATE COUGH SYRUP	117	635	1.11	39.2	922	1.5	$82.98	$.13	.072
P-O-E-G-(FECAL SOFTENER)	113	627	1.10	40.3	1270	2.0	$63.50	$.10	.055
ACETYLSALICYLIC ACID ALBA,5GR.	102	604	1.06	41.3	1255	2.1	$75.30	$.12	.065
ANTI-BACTERIAL DETERGENT	144	604	1.06	42.4	1073	1.8	$128.76	$.21	.111
PHENOBARB 8MG EPHEDR 25MG THEOPHYL 120MG,LAC	PET	582	1.02	43.4	86052	147.9	$163.21	$.28	.141
ACETAMINOPHEN TABLETS, 300 MG. 40	101	573	1.01	44.4	1431	2.5	$572.40	$1.00	.493
BELLADONNA & PHENO- BARBITAL MIX (HOSP.FORMULA)	DNE	539	.95	45.4	165350	306.8	$61.00	$.11	.053
ALUMINUM HYD.MAGNESIUM HYD GEL 150 ML,SU	ALM	536	.94	46.3	5962	11.1	$387.49	$.72	.334
ANTITUSSIVE COUGH MIXTURE	115	519	.91	47.2	659	1.3	$125.21	$.24	.108
METHYLDOPA 250MG,MS	ALD	497	.87	48.1	90313	181.7	$4786.56	$9.63	4.126
DIPHENHYDRAMINE 50MG,PD	B50	492	.86	49.0	30236	61.5	$90.69	$.18	.078
DIAZEPAM 10MG	VL10	448	.79	49.7	32803	73.2	$1836.96	$4.10	1.584
CHLORPROPAMIDE 250MG	DB250	390	.68	50.4	62476	160.2	$4060.91	$10.41	3.501
PSEUDOEPHEDRINE 60MG,LL	SU60	380	.67	51.1	18468	48.6	$53.53	$.14	.046
CHLORDIAZEPOXIDE 25MG	L25	370	.65	51.7	33785	91.3	$1655.45	$4.47	1.427
TOLBUTAMIDE 500MG	O	353	.62	52.4	76512	216.7	$4208.15	$11.92	3.628
FERROUS SULFATE TABLETS,5 GR.	158	350	.61	53.0	501	1.4	$55.11	$.16	.048
TRIAMCINOLONE .1% CR,LAC	TMC.1	347	.61	53.6	54930	158.3	$1226.52	$3.53	1.057
MULTIPLE VITAMIN,TO	MVT	345	.61	54.2	38692	112.2	$100.53	$.29	.087
RESERPINE 0.25MG,KS	R.25	342	.60	54.8	46340	135.5	$23.16	$.07	.020
MILK OF MAGNESIA	111	332	.58	55.4	500	1.5	$110.00	$.33	.095
SACCHARIN TABLETS,1/4 GR.	163	329	.58	55.9	413	1.3	$165.20	$.50	.142
ASPIRIN COMPOUND TABLETS	104	325	.57	56.5	448	1.4	$49.28	$.15	.042
AMPICILLIN 250MG,SQ	AMP250	321	.56	57.1	14974	46.6	$913.40	$2.85	.787
LANOLIN AND COLD CREAM	149	309	.54	57.6	567	1.8	$45.36	$.15	.039
TRIHEXYPHENIDYL 2MG,SC	ART2	305	.54	58.2	20313	66.6	$81.23	$.27	.070
ERYTHROMYCIN 250MG,UP	ER	302	.53	58.7	12505	41.4	$889.09	$2.94	.766
SULFAMETHOXAZOLE 500MG	GL	299	.52	59.2	18794	62.9	$496.09	$1.66	.428
ISOPROTERENOL METERED AEROSOL,RK	ISUM	299	.52	59.7	896	3.0	$1075.19	$3.60	.927
NEEDLES(26X1/2'')REUSABLE	133	294	.52	60.3	446	1.5	$53.52	$.18	.046
SECOBARBITAL SODIUM 100MG,IG	SC100	289	.51	60.8	11595	40.1	$48.67	$.17	.042
ALCOHOL,ISOPROPYL,70%	127	286	.50	61.3	400	1.4	$32.00	$.11	.028

Table II. Prescriptions for Narcotic Drugs

DRUG	DATE	DOCTOR	QTY	DUR	PATIENT	PF#	RX#	PHARM
DIPHENOXYLATE 2.5 MG ATROPINE .025MG	691215	SAUR	200	-	JOHN L. FRANCIS	0	693490550	ALS
ASPIRIN 300MG CODEINE 30MG,BW	691201	STOFFORD	30	-	HENRY SANUDO	187188	693351552	JOH
ASPIRIN 300MG CODEINE 30MG,BW	691212	HENNING	30	-	HENRY SANUDO	187188	693461903	BEN
ASPIRIN 300MG CODEINE 30MG,BW	691211	MELGARD	50	-	ALBERTA MILLER CT	724362	693450165	PKC
ASPIRIN 300MG CODEINE 30MG,BW	691216	BOBO	100	17	ALBERTA MILLER	724362	693500122	BEN
ASPIRIN 300MG CODEINE 30MG,BW	691219	MOORE	100	13	ALBERTA MILLER	724362	693531270	YAS
ASPIRIN 300MG CODEINE 30MG,BW	691224	LEE	100	-	ALBERTA MILLER	724362	693580475	JOH
ASPIRIN 300MG CODEINE 30MG,BW	691201	MILGARD	24	2	JAMES ANDREWS	872403	693351392	DJT
ASPIRIN 300MG CODEINE 30MG,BW	691201	MILGARD	24	2	JAMES ANDREWS	872403	693351346	DJT
ASPIRIN 300MG CODEINE 30MG,BW	691209	CHOE	100	-	J. CARRILLO	883988	693430986	GML
ASPIRIN 300MG CODEINE 30MG,BW	691231	CHOE	100	8	JULIANA CARRILLO (HD	883988	693650057	BAC
ASPIRIN 300MG CODEINE 30MG,BW	691212	SELTZER	30	8	WILLARD PACE	1017748	693461442	RST
ASPIRIN 300MG CODEINE 30MG,BW	691230	KUNIMOTO	50	6	WILLARD PACE	1017748	693641508	ENG
ASPIRIN 300MG CODEINE 30MG,BW	691216	LEE	100	17	CRAWLEY WEBB	1061483	693500242	EPS
ASPIRIN 300MG CODEINE 30MG,BW	691217	LEE	50	8	CRAWLEY WEBB	1061483	693510237	PKC
ASPIRIN 300MG CODEINE 30MG,BW	691224	GREEN	100	17	CRAWLEY WEBB	1061483	693580597	DJT
ASPIRIN 300MG CODEINE 30MG,BW	691223	GOODRELL	12	-	ALICE JACKSON	1066655	693572216	LHH
ASPIRIN 300MG CODEINE 30MG,BW	691226	CORDOBA	25	4	ALICE JACKSON	1066655	693600434	RHS
ASPIRIN 300MG CODEINE 30MG,BW	691205	CORDOBA	40	7	JEANETTE ANTHONY	1129995	693390712	GML
ASPIRIN 300MG CODEINE 30MG,BW	691216	CORDOBA	30	2	JEANETTE ANTHONY	1129995	693500578	PKC
ASPIRIN 300MG CODEINE 30MG,BW	691205	EULIN	15	-	CLEVELAND MITCHELL	1193691	693391332	MDM
ASPIRIN 300MG CODEINE 30MG,BW	691212	TALL	12	2	CLEVELAND MITCHELL	1193691	693460564	MJD
DIPHENOXYLATE 2.5 MG ATROPINE .025MG	691206	VAUGHERY	200	33	LENA SAMPSON	1210437	693400569	ENG
ASPIRIN 300MG CODEINE 30MG,BW	691208	TALL	20	3	BILLY THOMPSON	1328683	693421328	RHS
ASPIRIN 300MG CODEINE 30MG,BW	691209	CORDOBA	15	3	BILLY THOMPSON	1328683	693431189	MJD
ASPIRIN 300MG CODEINE 30MG,BW	691210	FISHER	120	-	DORIS KELLY	1361073	693441829	RST
TERPIN HYDRATE CODEINE ELIXIR,LAC	691226	ADELBERG	240	6	DORIS KELLY	1361073	693600399	RHS
ASPIRIN 300MG CODEINE 30MG,BW	691217	TALL35320	12	2	FRANK GAMBOA	1372166	693510595	JOH
ASPIRIN 300MG CODEINE 30MG,BW	691223	TALL	12	2	FRANK GAMBOA	1372166	693570137	PKC
ASPIRIN 300MG CODEINE 30MG,BW	691203	TALL	20	3	PETE MARRUJO	1382164	693370631	YAS
ASPIRIN 300MG CODEINE 30MG,BW	691210	TALL	20	3	PETE MARRUJO	1382164	693440143	ALS
ASPIRIN 300MG CODEINE 30MG,BW	691223	SHERMAN	30	4	DALTON MC FRAZIER	1438665	693571415	PKC
ASPIRIN 300MG CODEINE 30MG,BW	691230	SHERMAN	25	4	DALTON MC FRAZIER	1438665	693640664	PKC
ASPIRIN 300MG CODEINE 30MG,BW	691203	GROVE	480	16	FRANK BLAKE	1547336	693370310	LMG
TERPIN HYDRATE CODEINE ELIXIR,LAC	691217	BROWNE	480	16	FRANK BLACK	1547336	693510619	RHS
ASPIRIN 300MG CODEINE 30MG,BW	691205	TALL	24	4	WHEELER CONWAY	1586493	693390562	MJD
ASPIRIN 300MG CODEINE 30MG,BW	691212	CORDOBA	12	2	WHEELER CONWAY	1586493	693460113	MJD
ASPIRIN 300MG CODEINE 30MG,BW	691203	BOBO	50	4	WM BEAVER	1722542	693370145	BEN
ASPIRIN 300MG CODEINE 30MG,BW	691209	UTTSINGER	35	3	WILLIAM BEAVER	1722542	693431591	RST
ASPIRIN 300MG CODEINE 30MG,BW	691216	SHPALL	50	8	WILLIAM BEAVER	1722542	693500642	BEN
ASPIRIN 300MG CODEINE 30MG,BW	691219	PAK	100	17	WILLIAM BEAVER	1722542	693531718	ENG
ASPIRIN 300MG CODEINE 30MG,BW	691203	BELLIN	24	2	BERNICE CLEMONS	1739791	693371717	GLS
ASPIRIN 300MG CODEINE 30MG,BW	691205	TALL	20	3	BERNICE CLEMONS	1739791	693391318	GLS
ASPIRIN 300MG CODEINE 30MG,BW	691209	TALL	20	3	BERNICE CLEMONS	1739791	693431659	RHS
ASPIRIN 300MG CODEINE 30MG,BW	691209	BILLIN	20	3	JOSEPH ARMSTRONG	1741859	693431920	GLS
ASPIRIN 300MG CODEINE 30MG,BW	691210	TALL	20	3	JOSEPH ARMSTRONG	1741859	693440623	RHS

(4) Reports on all prescriptions for dangerous drugs
     that exceed a defined amount or frequency.

(5) Reports on concurrent prescribing defined as inap-
     propriate.

(6) Reports on any drug item for individual prescriptions
     that exceed defined amounts, as shown in Table III.

(7) Reports on any drug item for multiple prescriptions
     that exceed a defined frequency of occurrence.

(8) Drug history by patient at the time of clinic visit for
     all prescriptions within a predetermined time inter-
     val.

(9) Inventory reports of amounts purchased and amounts
     dispensed.

(10) Listing of physicians and prescriptions written by
     these physicians.

(11) Listing by clinic area of prescriptions originating
     from this clinic area.

B. Displayed Reports

(1) Prescription drug history displayed upon request in
     clinic at time of patient visit. This includes pre-
     vious suspected adverse reactions and drugs obtained
     from sources outside the environment of Los Angeles
     County-USC Medical Center.

(2) Recall of drug codes.

(3) Recall of cost values.

C. Statistical Data Analysis of Prescribing Patterns

This is carried out periodically to assess any changes in
prescribing patterns associated with educational programs or
feedback of information to the prescribing physician. A detailed example of such a study is given in the next section.

Table III. Distribution of 4003 Drug Prescriptions for
L10., Chlordiazepoxide 10 MG from 6/24/69 to 11/07/69

QTY PRESCRIBED	# OF RX	% OF TOTAL # OF RX	CUM %	% OF TOTAL QTY	CUM %
5	1	.12 %	.12 %	.01 %	.01 %
10	8	.94 %	1.05 %	.12 %	.13 %
12	6	.70 %	1.75 %	.11 %	.23 %
15	6	.70 %	2.45 %	.14 %	.36 %
20	23	2.68 %	5.13 %	.67 %	1.03 %
21	1	.12 %	5.24 %	.04 %	1.06 %
24	3	.35 %	5.59 %	.11 %	1.16 %
25	16	1.87 %	7.46 %	.58 %	1.74 %
26	1	.12 %	7.57 %	.04 %	1.78 %
30	80	9.32 %	16.89 %	3.48 %	5.25 %
35	4	.47 %	17.35 %	.21 %	5.46 %
36	1	.12 %	17.47 %	.06 %	5.51 %
40	36	4.19 %	21.66 %	2.09 %	7.59 %
42	1	.12 %	21.77 %	.07 %	7.65 %
45	2	.24 %	22.01 %	.14 %	7.78 %
50	195	22.71 %	44.71 %	14.12 %	21.90 %
60	42	4.89 %	49.60 %	3.65 %	25.54 %
70	1	.12 %	49.71 %	.11 %	25.64 %
75	5	.59 %	50.30 %	.55 %	26.19 %
80	6	.70 %	50.99 %	.70 %	26.88 %
90	27	3.15 %	54.14 %	3.52 %	30.40 %
100	297	34.58 %	88.71 %	42.99 %	73.39 %
120	16	1.87 %	90.58 %	2.78 %	76.17 %
150	25	2.91 %	93.49 %	5.43 %	81.59 %
180	1	.12 %	93.60 %	.27 %	81.85 %
200	40	4.66 %	98.26 %	11.58 %	93.43 %
240	1	.12 %	98.38 %	.35 %	93.78 %
250	2	.24 %	98.61 %	.73 %	94.50 %
300	10	1.17 %	99.77 %	4.35 %	98.85 %
400	2	.24 %	100.00 %	1.16 %	100.00 %

TOTAL QTY PRESCRIBED = 69089   TOTAL # OF RX = 859   MEAN = 80.5   MEDIAN = 75.0   MODE = 100,

IV. A STUDY OF PRESCRIBING PATTERNS

A. Rationale

In recent years increasing interest has been focused on a new concept known as drug utilization review [5-8], a dynamic approach aimed at improving patient care by instituting a more rational use of drugs.

Rational drug therapy itself has been defined as the right drug for the right patient, at the right time, in the right amounts, with due consideration of cost [9]. Recent assertions that much modern prescribing is irrational [10] have not been seriously challenged.

The clinical need for rational prescribing has been stressed by numerous workers in such countries as Great Britain [11-18], the United States [7-9, 19-25], Canada [26, 27], and Norway [28]. The economic need has been similarly emphasized. With the growing concern over rapidly rising costs in the private practice of medicine, and under both private and governmental health insurance programs in Great Britain, the United States and other nations [29], rational drug therapy appears clearly essential in order to make optimum use of the health dollar.

In addition, as Dunlop noted in 1969 [30], elimination of the financial barrier by means of the British National Health Service greatly encouraged overprescribing and has resulted in the dispensing of "great quantities" of prescribed drugs which are not consumed but left in home medicine cupboards, contributing to the current epidemic of accidental or deliberate self-poisoning. Others have warned that similar overprescribing may contribute to the supply of amphetamines, barbiturates, and other drugs reaching illegitimate channels [31].

Whatever the basis for seeking more rational prescribing – whether for clinical reasons or economic reasons, or both

– it seems necessary that suitable drug-utilization review
procedures should be instituted wherever feasible. Such procedures can achieve success only if they are based on an understanding of the problem and the goals sought, and an agreement through peer judgment on those characteristics which
may signal irrational or inappropriate prescribing patterns.

In previous publications we have described the methods
by which we gathered, reviewed, and analyzed preliminary
data on certain prescribing patterns [1]. From the results
of those early studies it appears that remedial measures are
warranted [2]. In the present paper we are presenting additional data on inappropriate prescribing patterns by individual physicians, some of the characteristics of those physicians, and the cost represented by this type of therapy.

B. Methods

The Los Angeles County-University of Southern California
Medical Center is one of the largest hospitals in the world,
serving a patient population of approximately 1 million. In the
outpatient clinics alone, about 900 physicians each year write
about 600,000 prescriptions that are dispensed to 200,000 individuals. Two pharmacies – the Outpatient Pharmacy and
the Unit I Pharmacy – dispense essentially all prescriptions
for outpatients. The Outpatient Pharmacy dispenses all prescriptions for adults coming to the hospital on scheduled appointments. The Unit I Pharmacy processes all prescriptions for patients being discharged from the hospital and for
those treated in the Medical Center's emergency sections as
unscheduled patients.

Since November 1967 outpatient prescriptions at the Medical Center have been processed by computer techniques. The
use of these electronic data processing methods is an integral

part of the drug dispensing system; it does not involve any retrospective entry of data, with the inherent risk of errors stemming from insertion of information long after the fact.

Most of the patients receive their drugs without charge. For those who are billed, drug costs are included in a single bill which covers physician services, laboratory work, and other services and supplies.

In a preliminary analysis [2] it was found that the 78 most frequently prescribed drugs represented more than 80% of all outpatient prescriptions. As the data base for this study, 52,733 consecutive prescriptions dispensed to outpatients between June 24 and September 7, 1969, for these 78 drugs were analyzed to indicate the nature and frequency of certain undesirable prescribing patterns. In this study attention was directed toward three types of undesirable prescribing:

(1) Excessive drug quantities on an individual prescription. *

(2) Excessive amounts of an individual drug theoretically in the possession of a patient as the result of multiple or repeated prescriptions.

(3) Concurrent prescriptions of different drugs considered to be inappropriate because of the risk of undesirable drug interaction.

Other types of irrational prescribing, such as the prescription of a drug or dosage inappropriate for the intended purpose, or the prescription of an expensive drug product when a less costly product would be logically expected to give the same clinical effects, are currently under examination.

---

*These will be further refined when diagnostic information is correlated with the therapeutic agent.

The definitions of what does or does not represent excessive-quantity prescribing were developed by a group of five
physicians and two pharmacists, who worked for $1\frac{1}{2}$ years in
frequent consultation with representatives of all the major
specialties (e. g. , medicine, surgery, obstetrics, etc.) and
subspecialties (e. g. , dermatology, gastroenterology, cardi-
ology, etc.). The appropriate definitions were established
for each of the drug items listed on the Medical Center formulary for outpatient use, but not generally announced.

These definitions are admittedly arbitrary, but they are
based on the judgment and experience of the committee members and their advisors, and take into account such factors
as the crowded clinics, the heavy patient load of this particular hospital, the patients it serves, and the accepted practices of the community.

It is possible, at least in theory, that the limits set on
appropriate prescription quantities might be established so
arbitrarily that the judgments would be illogically rigid. Thus,
it might be ruled that a prescription calling for 100 tablets of
a particular drug would be considered appropriate, while one
calling for 101 tablets would be considered inappropriate.
Such a situation did not, in fact, arise. In those prescriptions
considered to be inappropriate, the prescribed amounts were
generally found to be substantially larger – two, three, five,
or even ten times larger - than the approved quantity.

Typical is the distribution of prescriptions for chlor-
diazepoxide- 10 mg (Fig. 3) with an assigned limit of 100
capsules. Of 4003 prescriptions, 2669 (66. 7%) were within
this limit, while 66 (1. 6%) exceeded it by 1-49%, 289 (7. 2%)
exceeded it by 50-99%, 703 (17. 6%) exceeded it by 100-199%,
217 (5. 4%) exceeded it by 200-299%, and 62 (1. 5%) exceeded
it by 300-700%.

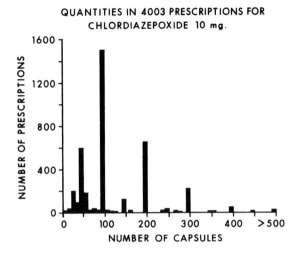

Fig. 3. Distribution of quantities requested in prescriptions for chlordiazepoxide.

C. Results

1. Undesirable Quantities – Individual Prescription

Of the 52,733 consecutive prescriptions, representing the 78 most frequently prescribed drug products for outpatients, there were 6844 (12.4%) that called for drug amounts in what were defined as excessive quantities. Table IV shows the defined limit in terms of numbers of tablets or capsules for the 30 most frequently prescribed drug products, together with the percentage of prescriptions exceeding this limit for each item, and the maximum quantity prescribed in any single prescription.

It is noteworthy that the percentage of excessive-quantity prescriptions was especially high in the case of frequently prescribed sedatives and tranquilizers – meprobamate-400 mg, 39.5%; chlordiazepoxide-10mg, 33.3%; diazepam-5 mg, 33.0%;

TABLE IV

Defined Limits for 30 Most Prescribed Drugs,
Percentage of Prescriptions Below and Above the Limit,
and the Maximum Quantity Prescribed

Drug product (strength in mg)	Total no. Rx's	Approved limits (no. caps or tabs)	No. Rx's under limit No.	%	No. Rx's over limit No.	%	Max. No. units prescribed in single Rx
1. Propoxyphene (65)	6673	300	6633	99.4	40	0.6	500
2. Hydrochlorothiazide (50)	5171	300	5126	99.1	45	0.9	600
3. Chlordiazepoxide (10)	4003	100	2669	66.7	1334	33.3	800
4. Diazepam (5)	2592	100	1737	67.0	855	33.0	600
5. Aspirin-codeine (300/30)	2319	100	2290	98.8	29	1.2	300
6. Digoxin (0.25)	2005	200	1977	98.6	28	1.4	400
7. Phenobarbital (30)	1515	200	1063	70.2	452	29.8	1300
8. Diphenylhydantoin (100)	1372	400	1201	87.5	171	12.5	1200
9. Methyldopa (250)	1340	350	1228	91.6	112	8.4	800
10. Chloral hydrate (500)	1261	100	1222	96.9	39	3.1	300
11. Chlorpropamide (250)	1153	300	1094	94.9	59	5.1	600
12. Diphenhydramine (50)	1139	100	987	86.7	152	13.3	800

13.	PET*	1053	200	828	78.6	225	21.4	1000
14.	Reserpine (0.25)	1041	300	1009	96.9	32	3.1	500
15.	Tetracycline (250)	984	100	909	92.4	75	7.6	500
16.	Chlorpheniramine (4)	919	100	801	87.2	118	12.8	600
17.	Tolbutamide (500)	917	300	787	83.6	150	16.4	750
18.	Sulfamethoxazole (500)	915	200	906	99.0	9	1.0	300
19.	Phenoxymethyl penicillin potassium (250)	836	50	781	93.4	55	6.6	400
20.	Thyroid (60)	688	600	666	96.8	22	3.2	1200
21.	Chlordiazepoxide (25)	677	100	477	70.5	200	29.5	794
22.	Nitroglycerine (0.4)	659	200	583	88.5	76	11.5	1000
23.	Multiple vitamins	653	200	617	94.5	36	5.5	400
24.	Meprobamate (400)	640	100	387	60.5	253	39.5	800
25.	Prednisone (5)	632	200	541	85.6	91	14.4	600
26.	Secobarbital sodium (100)	608	60	478	78.6	130	21.4	200
27.	Furosemide (40)	596	100	527	88.4	69	11.6	2000
28.	Trihexyphenidyl (2)	576	200	561	97.4	15	2.6	600
29.	Diazepam (10)	545	100	419	76.9	126	23.1	400
30.	Pseudoephedrine (60)	545	100	514	94.3	31	5.7	500

*PET – phenobarbital (8), ephedrine (25), theophylline (120).

phenobarbital-30mg, 29. 8%; isazepan-2 mg, 25. 9%; diazepan-
10 mg, 23. 1%; secobarbital sodium-100 mg, 21. 4%; and pheno-
barbital-15 mg, 20. 4%.

Table V shows the distribution of the excessive-quantity
prescriptions for these and other products involved most often
in this type of inappropriate prescribing.

It likewise seems noteworthy that these sedative or tran-
quilizing agents were involved in prescriptions written for
what would seem to be exceedingly large quantities. Thus,
prescriptions for meprobamate-400 mg and chlordiazepoxide-
10 mg, each with a defined limit of 100, were prescribed in
quantities as high as 800. For phenobarbital-30 mg, with a
limit of 200, prescriptions for as many as 1300 were found.

a. Physician Characteristics. The 52, 733 prescriptions analyzed here were written by 870 different physicians.
Of the 6844 inappropriate prescriptions, approximately 50%
were written by 30 physicians, or 3. 4% of the total (Fig. 4).
Table VI shows certain characteristics of these 30 physicians.

Most of these individuals were physicians hired solely for
the purpose of caring for outpatients. Seven of the 30 − including two interns − have been in practice for 1 year or less,
four for 2 years, and three for 3 years. Four of them, however, had been in practice for much longer periods − one for
20 years, one for 23 years, one for 24 years, and one for 36
years. One of the latter group was a specialist in internal
medicine, serving on the medical faculty.

Seven of the 30 physicians wrote 9179 prescriptions (17. 4%
of the total), of which 2365 called for drug amounts that exceeded the defined limits (37. 6% of all excessive-quantity prescriptions). The highest percentage of excessive-quantity
prescriptions written by any one physician was slightly more
than 50%.

No relationship was found between the percentage of inappropriate prescriptions and the total of prescriptions writ-

TABLE V

Distribution of Excessive-Quantity Prescriptions for 13 Selected Drug Items

Drug product (strength in mg)	Total No. Rx's	% with excess quant.	Appr. limit	No. of excessive-quantity prescriptions								
				101-200	201-300	301-400	401-500	501-600	601-700	701-800	801-900	901+
Meprobamate (400)	640	39.5	100	187	37	19	8	1	0	1	0	0
Chlordiazepoxide (10)	4003	33.3	100	1001	264	50	13	4	0	1	0	0
Diazepam (5)	2592	33.0	100	660	148	37	3	7	0	0	0	0
Phenobarbital (30)	1515	29.8	200	NA*	258	97	34	30	2	13	1	4
Chlordiazepoxide (25)	677	29.5	100	139	40	15	3	2	0	1	0	0
Allopurinol (100)	326	26.7	200	NA	69	10	6	1	0	0	0	1
Diazepam (2)	239	25.9	100	47	15	0	0	0	0	0	0	0
Phenoxymethol penicillin potassium (250)	274	24.1	300	NA	NA	64	2	0	0	0	0	0
Diazepam (10)	545	23.1	100	96	21	9	0	0	0	0	0	0
Amitriptyline (25)	261	22.2	200	NA	47	7	2	0	0	2	0	0
Secobarbital sodium (100)	608	21.4	60	-†								
PET‡	1053	21.4	200	NA	157	41	25	1	0	3	0	1
Phenobarbital (15)	418	20.6	200	NA	58	22	4	0	0	2	0	0

*NA - not applicable

†Number of excessive-quantity prescriptions: 61-120 units, 126 Rx's; 121-200 units, 4 Rx's.

‡PET - phenobarbital (8), ephedrine (25), theophylline (120).

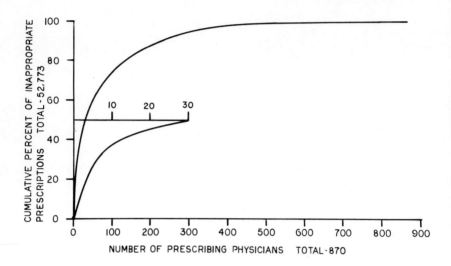

Fig. 4. Cumulative percentage of inappropriate prescriptions for defined excessive quantities plotted against the
number of individual prescribing physicians. The insert in
the lower left-hand corner magnifies the initial part of the
curve.

ten by an individual physician. For example, one so-called
"high prescriber" wrote 1096 prescriptions, of which 399
(36.4%) called for drugs in excessive amounts, but another
"high prescriber" wrote 1758 prescriptions, of which only 189
(10.8%) involved excessive amounts. In contrast, one "low
prescriber" wrote only 88 prescriptions, but 45 of these (51.1%)
were for excessive quantities.

Generally, when a physician wrote prescriptions for excessive quantities of one drug, he followed the same pattern
with other drugs. Among the 30 physicians with the highest
number of inappropriate prescriptions, all prescribed at least
11 different drug products in excessive amounts, while one
prescribed excessive quantities for 35 different products.

b. Costs. The total cost to the Medical Center for
the 52,733 prescriptions studied was $161,791. Twenty

TABLE VI

Some Characteristics of the 30 Physicians Accounting for the
Majority of the Excessive-Quantity Prescriptions

Physician	Years in pract.	Position*	Total no. Rx's written	Excessive-quantity Prescriptions No.	%	No. Drug product involved
A	6	-	88	45	51.1	21
B	7	-	170	80	47.1	16
C	36	-	235	88	37.4	15
D	8	-	1096	399	36.4	11
E	2	R	201	72	35.8	15
F	2	R	76	24	31.6	11
G	5	-	86	27	31.4	11
H	0	I	82	25	30.5	15
I	7	-	98	27	27.6	10
J	4	-	1305	347	26.6	35
K	24	-	1133	267	23.6	35
L	1	R	144	33	22.9	11
M	1	R	168	37	22.0	12
N	1	R	213	45	21.1	11
O	3	R	117	23	19.7	11
P	2	R	181	34	18.8	14
Q	4	R	118	22	18.6	11
R	4	R	110	20	18.2	11
S	1	-	1554	259	16.7	35
T	0	I	156	26	16.7	14
U	1	R	144	24	16.7	13
V	3	R	445	73	16.4	17
W	2	R	243	31	12.8	16
X	9	-	188	24	12.8	11
Y	20	-	1505	170	11.3	21

Physician	Years in prac.	Position*	Total no. Rx's written	Excessive-quantity Prescription		
				No.	%	Drug involved
Z	8	-	1758	189	10.8	24
AA	8	-	828	85	10.3	36
BB	23	-	285	20	7.0	11
CC	3	R	888	55	6.2	15
DD	5	R	406	24	5.9	11

*I = intern; R = resident.

products accounted for 80.3% of this amount, and one product – propoxyphene HCl – itself accounted for 13.1% (Table VII).

The cost of the prescriptions calling for what were defined as excessive quantities was $21,195, or 13.1% of the total. Twenty physicians (2.5%) accounted for 50% of the cost of these excessive quantities, and one physician alone accounted for 10% (Fig. 5).

2. Undesirable Quantities – Multiple Prescriptions

The second type of irrational prescribing pattern - excessive amounts of a drug theoretically in the possession of a patient as a result of multiple or repeated prescriptions for the same product – was found to involve only 1.7% of all prescriptions. This relatively low ratio, however, does not necessarily indicate that the problem is insignificant. Clearly involved here is the availability of excessive quantities, with the risk of accidental poisoning or suicide, as well as the possibility of diverting the excessive quantities into illegal channels.

3. Inappropriate Concurrent Prescribing

It is becoming increasingly apparent that certain drugs should generally not be prescribed for use at the same time by

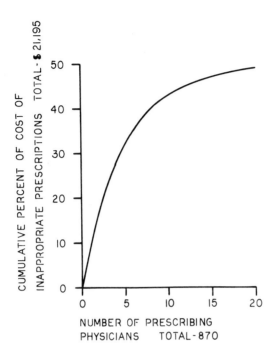

. Fig. 5. Cumulative percentage of drug cost of excessive drug quantities plotted against the number of prescribing physicians.

the same patient, because of the risk of drug interaction or other adverse reaction.

a. Drug Interaction. Because of potential drug inter-action, the concurrent prescription of certain products is con-sidered to be inappropriate. The following involve concurrent dispensing of products within a 7-day period for the same pa-tient during a consecutive 4-month period.

i. Methyldopa dispensed concurrently with dex-troamphetamine, ephedrine,or pseudoephedrine. Of 1261 pre-scriptions with dextroamphetamine, there were 29 with pheno-barbital-ephedrine-theophylline, and 16 with pseudoephedrine.

TABLE VII

The Cost of 20 Drug Products in Descending Order

Drug product (strength in mg)	Prescriptions* No.	Prescriptions* %	No. of units dispensed (caps or tabs)	Unit cost (in ¢)	Cost (in $)	% or total cost†
Propoxyphene (65) (Darvon)	6673	12.6	567,945	3.72	21,127.55	13.1
Chlordiazepoxide (10) (Librium)	4003	7.6	493,227	3.3	16,276.49	10.1
Chlorproamide (250) (Diabenase)	1153	2.2	201,351	6.5	13,087.82	8.1
Methyldopa (250) (Aldomet)	1340	2.5	239,369	5.3	12,683.38	7.8
Tolbutamide (500) (Orinase)	917	1.7	209,116	5.5	11,501.38	7.1
Diazepam (5) (Valium)	2592	4.9	301,058	3.8	11,444.02	7.1
Spironolactone (25) (Aldactone)	521	1.0	91,853	7.2	6,613.42	4.1
Hydrochlorothiazide (250) (Hydrodiuril)	5171	9.8	726,280	0.87	6,318.64	3.9
Acetazolamide (250) (Diamox)	312	0.6	80,135	5.17	4,142.98	2.6

Drug						
Chlordiazepoxide (25) (Librium)	677	1.3	83,193	4.9	4,076.46	2.5
Diazepam (10) (Valium)	545	1.0	55,673	5.6	3,117.69	2.0
Allopurinol (100) (Zyloprim)	326	0.6	59,653	5.2	3,101.96	1.8
Furosemide (40) (Lasix)	396	0.8	52,518	5.7	2,977.77	1.8
Indomethacin (25) (Indocin)	333	0.6	47,154	6.25	2,947.13	1.8
Nitrofurantoin (100) (Furadantin)	520	1.0	26,309	8.5	2,236.27	1.4
Aspirin-Codeine (300/30)	2319	4.4	78,753	2.69	2,184.46	1.4
Propantheline (15) (Probanthine)	398	0.8	70,370	2.7	1,899.99	1.1
Phenoxymethyl Penicillin Potassium (250)	836	1.6	29,129	5.9	1,718.61	1.1
Ampicillin (250)	382	0.7	19,549	6.1	1,192.49	0.7
Tetracycline (250)	984	1.9	58,296	1.95	1,136.77	0.7
Totals		57.6				80.3

*Total: 52,733 prescriptions for 78 most frequently prescribed drug products.

†Total cost: $161,791 for 52,733 prescriptions.

ii. Probenecid dispensed concurrently with aspirin. There were 299 prescriptions for probenecid. Of these, eight were dispensed with prescriptions for aspirin, and 10 with those for aspirin-codeine.

iii. Guanethidine dispensed concurrently with ephedrine, pseudoephedrine, or amitriptyline. Of 64 prescriptions for pseudoephedrine, there was one with ephedrine, three with phenobarbital-ephedrine-theophylline, and one with amitriptyline.

iv. Warfarin dispensed concurrently with phenobarbital. Prescriptions for warfarin totalled 283. Of these, 17 were prescribed concurrently with phenobarbital and five with phenobarbital-ephedrine-theophylline.

b. Drug Potentiation. In other instances, the concurrent prescription of two or more products is considered inappropriate because of the additive effect likely to result. The major types are the following.

i. Any two of the following: digoxin, digitalis, and digitoxin. There were 2005 prescriptions during the study period for digoxin. Of these, six were written concurrently with prescriptions for digitalis and two with those for digitoxin.

ii. Any two of the following: tolbutamide, chlorpropamide, and acetohexamide. There were 917 prescriptions for tolbutamide, of which 12 involved concurrent prescriptions for chlorpropamide and four for acetohexamide. There were also nine concurrent prescriptions for chlorpropamide and acetohexamide.

iii. Any two of the following: amitriptyline, imipramine, and nortriptyline. Of 261 prescriptions for amitriptyline, three were dispensed concurrently with those for imipramine and two with those for nortriptyline.

iv. Any two of the following: meprobamate, chlordiazepoxide, and diazepan. During the period of investigation

640 prescriptions for meprobamate were dispensed. Of these 29 were dispensed within 1 week* of prescriptions for chlordiazepoxide, and 49 concurrently with prescriptions for diazepam. In addition, there were 129 prescriptions for chlordiazepoxide dispensed within 1 week of prescriptions for diazepam. There were also 62 prescriptions for one dosage form of chlordiazepoxide accompanied by prescriptions for another dosage form of the same drug – usually written by different physicians – and 35 prescriptions of one dosage form of diazepam accompanied by concurrent prescriptions of a different form of the same product (Table VIII).

v. Any two of the following: chlorpromazine, trifluoperazine, and thioridazine. Of 430 prescriptions for chlorpromazine, 195 were dispensed concurrently with trifluoperazine and 11 with thioridazine. There were 43 prescriptions for trifluoperazine dispensed concurrently with prescriptions for thioridazine, and 18 prescriptions for one dosage form of thioridazine dispensed concurrently with prescriptions for a different dosage form of the same drug (Table IX).

vii. Any two of the following: phenobarbital-100 mg, secobarbital-100 mg, and pentobarbital-100 mg. Of 82 prescriptions for phenobarbital-100 mg, only two were dispensed concurrently with those for secobarbital-100 mg. Of 261 prescriptions for pentobarbital-100 mg, seven were dispensed concurrently with those for secobarbital-100 mg.

In general, this type of inappropriate prescribing was most frequently noted in the case of tranquilizers. The highest ratios of inappropriate concurrent prescriptions were 206

---

*In all instances, if the drug had been taken as directed there would have been at least a 2-week overlap with the defined inappropriate concurrent prescription.

TABLE VIII

Distribution of Inappropriate Concurrent Prescriptions:
Meprobamate, Chlordiazepoxide, and Diazepam*

	Meprobamate	Chlordiazepoxide			Diazepam		
	400 mg	5 mg	10 mg	25 mg	2 mg	5 mg	10 mg
Chlordiazepoxide – 5 mg	1	–					
Chlordiazepoxide – 10 mg	24	18	–				
Chlordiazepoxide – 25 mg	4	2	42	–			
Diazepam – 2 mg	2	0	3	1	–		
Diazepam – 5 mg	32	3	78	7	6	–	
Diazepam – 10 mg	15	1	26	10	1	28	–

*In number of prescriptions, 7-day period.

TABLE IX

Distribution of Inappropriate Concurrent Prescriptions:
Chlorpromazine, Thioridazine, and Tribluoperazine*

	Thioridazine				Trifluoperazine		
	10 mg	25 mg	50 mg	100 mg	2 mg	5 mg	10 mg
Chlorpromazine – 25 mg	0	0	0	0	2	2	0
Chlorpromazine – 30 mg	0	0	0	0	0	2	0
Chlorpromazine – 50 mg	0	1	1	1	9	22	20
Chlorpromazine – 75 mg	0	0	0	0	1	3	2
Chlorpromazine – 100 mg	0	2	0	5	8	31	29
Chlorpromazine – 150 mg	0	0	1	0	1	14	13
Chlorpromazine – 200 mg	0	0	0	0	0	7	21
Chlorpromazine – 300 mg	0	0	0	0	0	1	7
Thioridazine – 10 mg	—	1	0	0	0	1	0
Thioridazine – 25 mg		—			3	4	2
Thioridazine – 50 mg		13	—		1	8	6
Thioridazine – 100 mg			4	—	0	13	5

*In number of prescriptions, 7-day period.

(47. 9%) of 430 prescriptions for chlorpromazine, 238 (36. 8%) of 647 prescriptions for trifluoperazine, 72 (26. 3%) of 647 prescriptions for thioridazine, 78 (12. 2%) of 640 prescriptions for meprobamate, 213 (6. 8%) of 3137 prescriptions for diazepam and 220 (4. 7%) of 4680 prescriptions for chlordiazepoxide. Also among the high ratios was that for warfarin — 22 (7. 8%) of 283 prescriptions.

In the majority of cases, this kind of irrational prescribing concerned an individual patient receiving prescriptions from two or more physicians. Whether or not each of the physicians concerned here was aware that his patient was under the care of another physician at the same time has not been determined. Similarly, it is not known how many of these apparently inappropriate concurrent prescriptions had been cancelled, or the treatment otherwise altered, by verbal instructions to the patient. These subjects will be analyzed in further studies.

D. Discussion

The prescription of drugs in excessive quantities portrays on-going patterns actually used by physicians in the Medical Center. They do not represent conscious or unconscious violations of hospital regulations in this respect, since no such regulations were formally established and disseminated to members of the clinical staff. The data thus indicate the degree of excessive prescribing in this one large institution which occurred during a $2\frac{1}{2}$-month period without any degree of formal control.

From these records supporting our earlier view that tranquilizers, sedatives, analgesics, and other drug products are likely to be prescribed and dispensed in very large quantities, it would appear that some degree of control might well be instituted — in part to reduce the unjustifiable expenditure of funds, and in part to limit the risk of accidental or deliberate poisoning or the amount of these drugs moving into illicit channels.

To implement any effective control methods, at least three steps are essential

(1) There must be widespread agreement among the clinical staff that such an approach is both clinically and economically necessary.

(2) There must be complete or at least widespread agreement on the limits of each major drug product that may be rationally prescribed. In this connection, of course, it is essential that adequate provisions be made to permit the prescription of apparently excessive quantities under exceptional circumstances.

(3) There must be an adequate computer system or other method of data processing to make available to each prescriber (a) the approved maximum quantity for each drug and (b) the complete and up-to-date drug prescription record of each patient treated in the Medical Center.

It is obvious that such a program could not be readily utilized in the case of outpatients who are under the simultaneous treatment of two or more nonhospital-based physicians or who are in a position to have their prescriptions filled by nonhospital pharmacies that are not linked to a central computer system. For such an institution as the Los Angeles County-USC Medical Center, however, with drugs prescribed almost exclusively by hospital staff physicians and dispensed by hospital pharmacies, the use of this approach would seem to be both practical and essential. Steps leading to establishment of this system in the Medical Center are now underway.

It must be emphasized that the system should be designed
in such a manner that each physician is apprised within a matter of a few seconds or minutes – a time which is within reach
with the use of electronic techniques – of (1) the drug record
of the patient, including any reported drug allergies, (2) the
prescriptions for this patient which have been dispensed within the preceding weeks or months, (3) the peer judgment on
the maximum number of tablets or capsules of any product
which may be rationally dispensed at one time or over any
given period, and (4) those concurrent prescriptions which
present a risk of additive or synergistic reactions. As an
additional feature, the data processing system could be designed to indicate alternative dosage forms or other products
which might be used in place of the proposed drug to give the
same clinical results with less chance of adverse reaction or
at lower cost to the patient or the hospital.

In any case, it appears essential that the physician, once
he has been alerted to possible risks or needless expenditures,
must maintain his responsibility for making the final prescribing decision.

E. Summary

As a first step in controlling irrational prescribing, three
types of undesirable or inappropriate prescriptions have been
defined and identified by physicians and pharmacists at the
Los Angeles County-University of Southern California Medical
Center. These types are (1) excessive drug quantities specified in individual prescriptions, (2) undesirably frequent
prescriptions for the same drug, and (3) inappropriate concurrent prescriptions for different drugs.

Of 52,733 consecutive prescriptions for the 78 drug products most frequently dispensed to outpatients, representing

more than four-fifths of all outpatient prescriptions, it was found that 12.4% represented excessive-quantity prescriptions.

Most frequently involved were sedatives and tranquilizers. As many as 1300 tablets of one such agent were dispensed to one patient on a single prescription.

Of a prescribing population of about 800 physicians, 30 accounted for about 50% of these excessive-quantity prescriptions, and 20 of them accounted for about 50% of the cost of the excessive quantities.

No relationship was observed between the number of prescriptions written by a physician and the number of prescriptions for quantities considered excessive.

Only 1.7% of all prescriptions were considered to involve too frequent prescribing of the same drug, by either the same physician or different physicians. As part of this study, however, analysis of patient drug records showed that some outpatients were receiving as many as 54 prescriptions (12 on a single day), and as many as 7416 tablets or capsules of various drug products, over a 112-day period.

Numerous examples were found of concurrent prescriptions of two different drug products which could result in serious drug interaction or potentiation. Most frequently involved were prescriptions for sedatives and tranquilizers.

It is suggested that these types of irrational prescribing may be controlled in a medical center or hospital environment. This would require (1) agreement among the clinical staff that such an approach is both clinically and economically necessary (2) agreement through peer judgment on the limits of each major drug product that may be rationally prescribed (with provisions to permit the prescription of apparently excessive quantities under exceptional circumstances) and (3) the availability of an adequate computer system or other method of data processing.

The physician, once he has been alerted to possible risks or needless expenditures, must maintain his responsibility for making the final prescribing decision.

V. CONCLUSION

We have demonstrated the feasibility of a drug data center which can combine review procedures with the development of administrative policies. The policies that guide the hospital administration in relation to drug utilization within the environment have been influenced by the flexibility and availability of our prescription data. On the other hand, a mass of prescription data without well thought out definitions and policies requires the collaborative effort of physicians, pharmacists, nurses, and hospital administrators. These concepts are of more than local interest. The capability of combining review procedures with drug claims processing on a national level should favorably influence medical care standards.

ACKNOWLEDGMENTS

This work is supported in part by the Department of Health, Education, and Welfare, Office of the Secretary (Contract HEW-OS-70-89) and in part by the Social Security Administration (Contract number 467).

We are deeply indebted to Dr. Milton Silverman, University of California, San Francisco Medical Center, for his advice and help in the writing of this manuscript; to our electronic data processing programming staff, particularly Douglas Burks, Phyllis Licht, and Pamela Bailey; and to Mr. Jack Katzoff, pharmacist, Dr. Ronald Markman, and Dr. Mildred Milgrom for their contributions to this work.

REFERENCES

1. S. Seibert, S. Brunjes, J. C. Soutter, and R. F. Maronde, "Utilization of Computer Equipment and Technique in Prescription Processing," Drug Intelligence, 1, 342 (1967).

2. R. F. Maronde, D. Burkes, P. V. Lee, P. Licht, M. M. McCarron, M. McCary, and S. Seibert, "Physician Prescribing Practices; a Computer Based Study," Am. J. Hosp. Pharmacy, 26, 566 (1969)

3. ·American Medical Association, Utilization Review, American Medical Association, Chicago, Illinois, 1956, p. 116.

4. Avedis Donabedian, Milbank Memorial Fund Quarterly, 44, Part w, 166 (1966).

5. J. D. Wallace, Hospitals, 41, 70 (1967).

6. D. Slone, L. F. Gaetano, L. Lipworth, S. Shapiro, G. P. Lewis, and H. Jick, Public Health Reports, 84, 39 (1969).

7. U. S. Department of Health, Education, and Welfare, Task Force on Prescription Drugs, "Approaches to Drug Insurance Design," U. S. Government Printing Office, Washington, D. C., 1969, p. 640.

8. T. D. Rucker, "Drug Utilization Review," Amer. J. Hospital Pharmacy (in press).

9. U. S. Department of Health, Education, and Welfare, Task Force on Prescription Drugs, "The Drug Prescribers," U. S. Government Printing Office, Washington, D. C., 1968, p. 3.

10. U. S. Department of Health, Education, and Welfare,
     Task Force on Prescription Drugs, "Final Report,"
     U. S. Government Printing Office, Washington, D. C.,
     1969, p. 21.

11. J. P. Martin, Social Aspects of Prescribing, Heinemann,
     London, 1957, p. 73.

12. C. W. M. Wilson, J. A. Banks, R. E. A. Mapes, and
     S. M. T. Korte, British Medical J., 2, 604 (1963)

13. J. A. H. Lee, Proc. Royal Society of Medicine, 57, 1041
     (1964).

14. J. A. H. Lee, P. A. Draper, and M. Weatherall, Milbank
     Memorial Fund Quarterly, 43, 285 (1965).

15. C. W. M. Wilson, J. A. Banks, R. E. A. Mapes, and
     S. M. T. Korte, "The Assessment of Prescribing: A
     Study in Operational Research," in Problems and Pro-
     gress in Medical Care: Essays on Current Research
     (G. McLachlan, ed.), Oxford University Press, London,
     1964, p. 173.

16. C. W. M. Wilson, J. A. Banks, R. E. A. Mapes, and
     S. M. T. Korte, British Medical J., 2, 599 (1963).

17. C. R. B. Joyce, J. M. Last, and M. Weatherall, British
     J. Preventive and Social Medicine, 22, 170 (1968).

18. Sainsbury, Report of the Committee of Enquiry into the
     Relationship of the Pharmaceutical Industry with the
     National Health Service, Her Majesty's Stationery Office,
     London, 1967.

19. Paul Talalay, Drugs in Our Society, Johns Hopkins
     Press, Baltimore, 1964.

20. D. L. Azarnoff, D. B. Hunninglake, and J. Wortman,
     J. Chronic Diseases, 19, 1256 (1966).

21. L. E. Cluff, Hospital Practice, 2, 101 (1967)

22. Leslie J. DeGroot, (ed.), Medical Care, C. C. Thomas,
     Springfield, Illinois, 1967, p. 207.

23. Charlotte F. Muller, Amer. J. Public Health, 57, 2121
     (1967).

24. D. L. Wilbur, Proceedings of the Western Pharmacol-
     ogy Society, 11 (1968).

25. P. D. Stolley, and L. Lasagna, J. Chronic Diseases, 22,
     395 (1969).

26. R. E. Ogilvie, and J. Ruedy, Canadian Medical Assoc.
     J., 97, 1450 (1967).

27. Special Committee of the House of Commons on Drug
     Costs and Prices, "Second (Final) Report, " House of
     Commons, Canada, Queen's Printer and Controller of
     Stationery, Ottawa, Canada, 1967.

28. K. Evang, Health Service, Society and Medicine, Oxford
     University Press, London, 1960, p. 1250.

29. U. S. Department of Health, Education, and Welfare,
     Task Force on Prescription Drugs, "Current American
     and Foreign Programs, " U. S. Government Printing
     Office, Washington, D. C. , 1968.

30.   D. M. Dunlop, Annals of Internal Medicine, 71, 237
      (August 1969).

31.   M. Kreig, Black Market Medicine, Prentice-Hall,
      Englewood Cliffs, New Jersey, 1967.

4

On-Line Data Bank for Admissions, Laboratories and Clinics

Gene E. Thompson
Chief, Hospital Information Systems, Dept. of Hospitals
County of Los Angeles, Los Angeles, California

I. LOS ANGELES COUNTY DATA BANK DEFINITION

A. Introduction

The Los Angeles County Department of Hospitals operates one of the largest systems of patient care in the world. The system includes 9 hospitals with a total of over 6000 beds and a medical staff of over 2000 physicians. The initiation and maintenance of computer-based files on this enormous number of patients has created some special problems. This chapter summarizes the experience gained to date in the continuing development of this centralized data bank with approximately 80 on-line data terminals in 9 hospitals.

The admissions system is described, and the techniques used to identify patients are described.

B. Functional Parts of the Data Bank

The Los Angeles County Patient Data Bank was intended to provide a generalized framework for the collection of all data on patients who received either treatment of consultation in the Los Angeles County hospital system. This necessitated design in a relatively generalized manner to permit growth and development.

111

Although defining a somewhat specific group of patients who have contacted the Los Angeles County hospital system, we did not specify exactly the purpose of the data file, intending that this purpose might change or be augmented as time and opportunity permitted. This plan generally still remains effective. However, as with any plan, the methods have been better defined as time has progressed and experience has been gained.

In defining the functional parts of the Data Bank as it now exists for Los Angeles County hospitals, we use the concept of the "active" versus the "historical" record. Typically, the "active" portion shows extreme change during the period of time that the patient utilizes the hospital. It involves a large number of in-hospital systems and results in a number of byproduct reports and long-term data production. Typically, the active record contains a great amount of detail which has a very limited useful life.

We define the records themselves as functional collections of specifically oriented modules. For the logical design of the file, the records need have only a logical connection. In the case of the Los Angeles County patient records, this is accomplished by a master linking number between all modules of the records. Through this device we may have segments of the same logical record structure on different physical devices, such as disk, data cell, and magnetic tape, so that we may utilize the appropriate type of storage device according to the activity level and required retrieval time. We need this feature primarily for economy, since the more rapid retrieval devices also have a larger price tag.

The modules now existing and functional for the individual records of the patient data bank we call: the Identification module, which uniquely identifies each record and condenses

the identification factors which have the function of linking
the other record modules to a person; the Social and Financial
History module, the Urgent Medical History module; and the
Laboratory Data module. In the process of development we
have a Pharmacy Data module, a Clinical Data module, and
refinements of the Laboratory Data module as an Anatomical
Laboratory Data module, and a Chemical Laboratory Data
module.

The record module structure currently permits up to 16
types and 16 varieties of modules from different physical data
locations. The file needs this last provision because in some
cases later data do not obviate earlier data as, for instance,
a record of removal of a kidney does not obviate records relating to treatment for heart disease.

C. Mandatory Characteristics of a Data Bank

A data bank must have certain characteristics in order to
function properly. First, the file structure must have the
capability of expansion to cover the entire universe of data
for which it is designed. In the specific case of the patient
data bank, this would mean that any patient could fit into this
record structure regardless of which hospital, clinic, or
specialized service he had used.

The second mandatory characteristic of the data bank is
that the structure must be capable of receiving any information
applicable to its basic objectives. This does not mean that
records have been designed for all possible data, but rather
that new types of data can be incorporated without completely
redesigning the file.

The third mandatory characteristic of the data bank is
that a variety of levels of both entry and retrieval of data be
possible.

D. Optional Characteristics of a Data Bank

An optional characteristic is the capability of cross-
referencing data so that correlations between the various
segments of data may be derived. The structure of the data
bank provides the opportunities to make such correlations,
since we assume that all data relevant to a specific person or
object is automatically updated in the same location as all
other data for the person.

Another optional characteristic is universal standardization
of terminology. This is certainly a desirable characteristic
and would be necessary to correlate various records. However, it must be emphasized that data can be collected in
various forms and still be utilized by specific areas within
the data bank context without standardization being a necessary
prerequisite.

II. LOS ANGELES COUNTY HOSPITALS DATA BANK

The prime objective in development of the data bank for
Los Angeles County hospitals was that the system be oriented
to improve patient care. The data bank offered a significant
opportunity in this area by eliminating duplication of patient
data and by making a reliable current patient record available
at the point of contact with the patient.

For flexibility of development the simplest possible
techniques were employed. At the same time, the great
values inherent in centralized collection of data were recognized
and it was decided to set up a structure which would take
advantage of these values, if not immediately, then in the
eventual development. For this reason the central computer
center was located in the largest of the County hospitals, the
Los Angeles County-USC Medical Center (see Fig. 1a).

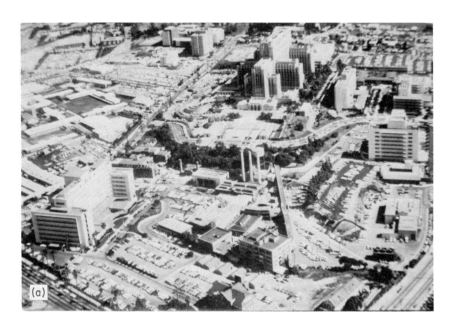

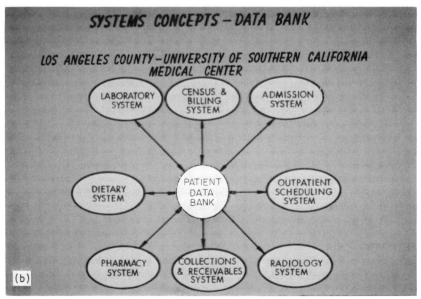

Fig. 1. (a) Aerial View of LAC-USC Medical Center,
looking south. (b) Data bank concept - modular systems with
a single data base.

A. Initial Structure

The initial modular structure for the data bank was chosen on very general terms. It was assumed that modules could be developed with relative independence and that the specific systems development effort could run in parallel with the development of programs to handle each module (see Fig. 1b). Over a period of time this initial record structure has been heavily altered.

Some general categories, such as laboratory data, have been broken into more specific categories. Experience has shown that anatomical pathology data does not fit alongside chemistry data. This is also true in the area of radiology, as radiation therapy data does not fit into the same context as x-ray data. This continued process of more specific identification probably will continue until the record structure is in close accord with the actual structure of data within the hospitals.

B. Cross-Reference Files

Cross-reference files between one segment of a record or file and another are very important in our system. In actual practice the development of such files is a specialized technique, which is being used exclusively for Los Angeles County. As new data elements are added to the files, the interrelationship with previously established data is done by cross referencing.

The difficulty with such a method is that it creates extra files to be updated every time an action is taken. It is not enough to update the basic patient file, the cross-reference file pointers must also be updated. The resulting files are longer but the technique allows great flexibility, which partially compensates for the format and content between

separate hospitals and separate functional areas within
hospitals. For example, a hospital which may select factors
for an urgent medical history which are different from those
selected by a second hospital. Through the cross-referencing
technique it is possible to interpret and mask these differences
automatically.

III. MODULAR RECORD TECHNIQUES

A. Multidirectional Expansion

Modular record techniques are the key to development of
a production data bank system. It is necessary to recognize
that any hospital data system must allow for expansion, including (1) geographic expansion, (such as adding new hospital
locations and new locations within the hospitals where data is
collected and patients are identified,) and, (2) expansion by
collection of additional types of data (viz., the addition of
radiology data on patients already in the system).

B. Partial Records and Partial Files

It must be recognized that for the foreseeable future,
the modular technique must be employed for records with
only partial data. In the present day hospital, it is simply
not possible to obtain a complete data collection on every
patient and every visit.

IV. DATA INPUT

A. Design Control

The control of the design of the data input system must
be resident with the hospital. Specific kinds of data input and
controls should be the province of the people who will actually
be doing the preparation. The data processing systems
designers have no particular problem thinking of new methods,
but they are definitely not qualified to specify input methods

in detail. The practical working answer to this is that the
first rough design should be presented to the hospital personnel
by the systems designers, but that it should be assumed that
several phases of redesign will be needed before the final
design is approved.

B. Installation and Feedback

Various alternatives can be chosen for data input. The
Los Angeles County system is based on using source data
collection by collecting the data as near the person originating
it as possible. The data processing alternatives are many,
but they fall into two main classes. One is terminal entry,
which refers to the use of any device which prepares computer-
readable data at the location where it is generated. This
includes such devices as paper-tape producing typewriters
and on-line video terminals. The second method is the
classical one of remote data preparation for centralized
conversion to computer-readable form. The oldest such
method, of course, is key punching with newer methods
available such as optical character recognition. Any method
of centralized data conversion represents a bottleneck and
the resulting collection of source documents and their conversion creates severe control problems. In our opinion, the
most desirable method is that of terminal entry, but the cost
of such installations may turn out to be prohibitive.

V.   ON-LINE SYSTEMS

A. Convenience versus Cost

Real-time processing is popular in the medical area
because of its convenience. In many locations where patient
care is rendered, it is possible to have at least a portion of
the capability of the computer present to assist the staff.
This convenience can, of course, be overstated, since intro-

ducing a computer as an element in patient care usually adds
a step above and beyond current practice. Many vaunted
hospital information systems have foundered on the rock of
resistance of doctors, nurses, and other patient-care
personnel who find the mechanics of entry and retrieval
neither convenient nor speedy enough for their needs. However, part of this problem is simply one of technological
development, and as more convenient hospital and patient-
care remote terminals are developed, it can be assumed that
this problem will be overcome.

A more serious factor to consider is the extremely high
base cost plateau which is necessary to mount even the most
basic real-time teleprocessing system. A major cost arises
from the minimum-size requirement of the central processing
unit. Systems under 128K words of core memory are
relatively rare, and most typical systems use 256K as well
as the relatively expensive disk or drum storage which is
required if rapid file access is to be achieved. General
purpose processors in this class will run from $17,000 to
$27,000 in monthly rental. Unit rental on disk storage runs
in the neighborhood of $1100-$5000 per month for the typical
configuration now being used. Beyond this we need a line
controlling unit running from $500 to $1100 per month, the
necessary transmission lines and the "modems", the decoding
and encoding devices at each end of the line. Then, of course,
there is the terminal itself which will run in the neighborhood
of $100 up to $500 a month. Add to this the personnel costs
for the installation and maintenance of the specialized teleprocessing software and the high cost of leaving the central
processing unit relatively free so that it can respond to in-
quiries quickly, and you begin with a very high-cost system.
It should be reasonably obvious, therefore, that only the

larger organizations can afford to set up this sort of system;
smaller groups will be compelled to go to one of the
commercial time-sharing companies, which is in itself an
expensive proposition.

There is a tremendous need to make on-line, real-time
teleprocessing facilities available despite the cost difficulties
because of the potential of better patient care through more
effective interdepartmental communications.

VI. ROLE OF TELEPROCESSING

A. Terminals

Currently available terminal units have the advantage of
several years of operational experience built into them.
Terminal reliability at this time is comparatively high, even
within environments which are neither air conditioned nor
humidity controlled. Existing terminals also generally have
many more features than are ordinarily used since they were
designed for the general market. As a result, it is possible
to use them in a number of different roles without specializing
the engineering characteristics or spending a great deal of
time worrying about the exact configuration.

There are some special shortcomings related to the fact
that existing terminals generally were designed to be used by
specifically trained operators, and, therefore, some of their
features are difficult to use by the casual operator. Also,
existing terminals tend to be bulky, and this is a definite draw-
back in view of the limited space availability within many
hospitals.

B. Terminal Interaction

It is possible to use terminals interacting with the system
in a number of different ways. The terminals can serve as

pure entry points, collecting data from on-going operations, storing that data, and manipulating it for later utilization. It is also possible for terminals to serve as a question-and-answer point, in effect allowing the operator of the terminal to converse with the computer files. On a higher level of sophistication, the terminal can be used in a general support of the overall computer facilities, up to and including writing and executing computer programs. It is important to recognize that the use of the terminal must be understood before the system to support that terminal is designed, since, in many cases, the system will alter radically as the uses change.

Figures 2 and 3 show the terminal system at the Los Angeles County - USC Medical Center.

VII.   CLINIC INFORMATION SYSTEM

A.   Clinic Schedule

One of the systems which is instrumental in the building of the data bank, but has an additional and equally important purpose, is the clinic information system. Relative to the operation of the data bank this system is the other half of the operation of the hospital. Patients treated in the clinic system will not be entering the normal inpatient admissions. Therefore, the analogous event to admission must be captured on the clinical side. This is the clinic visit. Capturing this event requires that clinic scheduling be undertaken. Clinic scheduling has proved to be a pitfall in many automated systems for hospitals.

A clinic schedule involves several possible levels of complexity. The basic scheduling function is extremely difficult because the clinics form a large number of entities, each with their own characteristics. Also, clinic scheduling is made very rigorous by the short time span involved in a

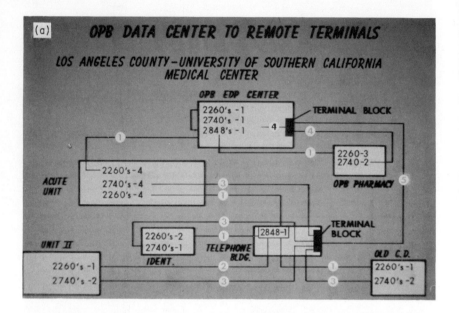

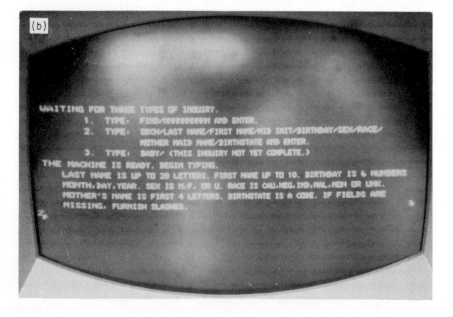

Fig. 2. (a) Initial cabling diagram for first set of terminals at LAC-USC Medical Center. (b) Close view of CRT
terminal display showing beginning display with instructions.

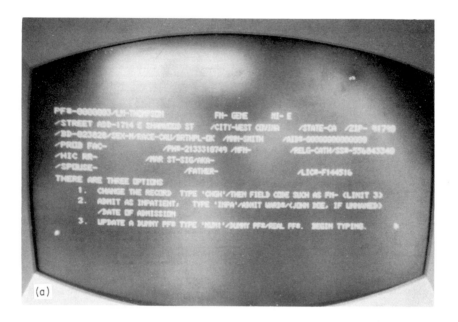

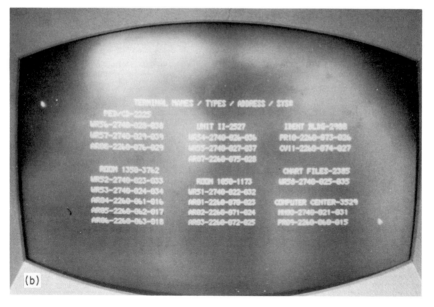

Fig. 3. (a) Close view of CRT terminal display showing
typical ident record format, plus instructions. (b) Close view
of CRT terminal display showing systems readout of terminal
locations by location, systems number - terminal type.

clinic visit. If you miss an inpatient on the way in, you will
catch up with him in the ward. If you miss a clinic patient
on his way in, he will be gone before you can do anything
about it. From the beginning, the registering procedure,
factor of physician selection, coordination of specialized
facilities such as laboratory tests required with the clinic,
coordination of multiple clinic visits and distribution of the
time spent in the various clinics and the different types of
therapy involved can all be designed and entered into the
computerized scheduling process.

B. Clinic Facilities Management

The byproduct of computerized scheduling is the more
effective management of clinic facilities. In clinic visit
scheduling it is possible to study and relate patient scheduling
from the collected data to the number of physicians needed,
number of examining rooms, preparation of laboratory
facilities, x-ray schedule, pharmacy loading, and other related internal facilities. If this data can be used to make
more effective utilization of the clinics resources then cost
savings may be realized.

C. Clinic Data Bank Characteristics

Clinic patients can create problems in the construction
of the data bank because, unlike inpatients, clinic patients
do not have a hard core of universally collected data. The
difference between outpatients in a psychiatry clinic and a
diabetic clinic is much greater than the difference between
a psychiatric outpatient and a psychiatric inpatient. For
this reason, the development of the data bank for outpatients
required greater flexibility in the modular design.

Another consideration in outpatients' clinic scheduling
is the very large numbers of people who are involved with

outpatient operations. Because the clinics often are operated
as completely separate entities, communication with involved
hospital personnel becomes of primary importance. As
opposed to admissions processing where a relatively small
select group performs the main work of admissions and the
patients are essentially funneled through special areas for
admission, out-patient clinics typically have multiple points
of admission and virtually everybody is involved in one way
or another with the scheduling and treatment of the patient.

VIII. ADMISSIONS SYSTEM

A. Admissions System Characteristics

The starting point for on-line real-time teleprocessing
in the Los Angeles County hospital system was the admissions
service at its largest hospital, the Los Angeles County - USC
Medical Center. The selection of this service for the beginning system was decided by three basic circumstances.

First, the Los Angeles County Department of Hospitals
has a typical method of patient admissions. It is required
that all patients be examined in an admitting area prior to
admission. This in effect creates a situation where all
admissions are emergencies since there is no preadmission
procedure. It also insures that if one can capture or review
data at the point of admission, virtually 100% of all patients
will be entered in the system.

The second circumstance was that the hospital in which
the initial system was to be established was so large that it
was practically impossible to start with an assumption of remote terminals on the wards. The Los Angeles County - USC
Medical Center has 2100 licensed beds and 110 wards.

Third, the immediate problem to be solved in the Los
Angeles County - USC Medical Center was one of improving

the admissions procedures to reduce the waiting time for
patients being examined and to provide the best possible
history data to the examining physicians. This is obviously
necessary since the admissions procedures virtually
guaranteed that the patient would be unknown to the examining
doctor. Therefore, the most practical medical history data
were to be provided (see Fig. 4 and 5).

B. File Basis

The file basis for the Los Angeles County Department
of Hospitals is that of the individual patient and the entire
data bank rests on individual patient records. This is not
the only basis on which a data bank can be built; some
alternatives would be family grouping, treatment grouping,
geographic grouping, or any generally usable criteria which
can be systematically and universally applied. The basis
must insure that in 100% of the cases, if there is a slot for
the patient, some minimum amount of information will also
be present and this information can be related to all other
pieces of data which will be added to it later. The processing
of admissions is designed to capture just this minimal part
of the data. In the system design for Los Angeles County, by
capturing each patient at the point of admission, it is assured
that there will be a minimal record available called the "Ident"
module to which all other data can relate.

C. Identification of Records

One of the key problems in any file is that the identifier
for current file records must be unique, or the file cannot be
maintained. The manual procedure previously used was based
on a Soundex Retrieval which brought together like-sounding
names and a history proven system of secondary identifying
factors. These factors, proven by years of hospital use,

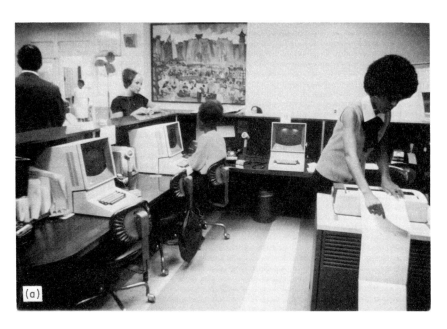

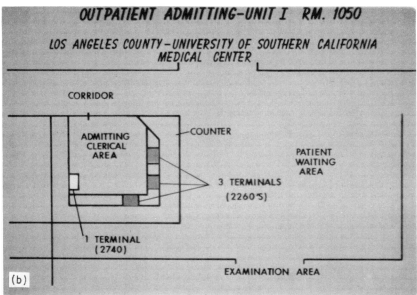

Fig. 4. (a) Interior view of clerical area with computer
terminals, Room 1050 Outpatient Admissions Area, LAC-USC
Medical Center. (b) Diagram of terminal placement in
clerical area of Room 1050, Outpatient Admissions Area,
LAC-USC Medical Center.

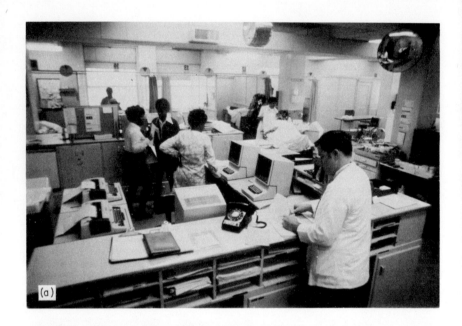

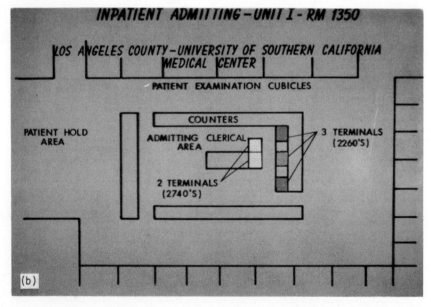

Fig. 5. (a) Interior view of clerical area with computer terminals, Room 1350, Main Inpatient Admitting Room, LAC-USC Medical Center. (b) Diagram of terminal placement in clerical area of Room 1350, Main Inpatient Admitting Room, LAC-USC Medical Center.

included the first and last name of the patient, address, state
of birth, date of birth, mother's maiden name, father's first
name, last name, age, sex, and race. The same factors
were used for identification in the computer system. The key
is the patient file number which is also correlated with the
social security or HI number for the patient. Numbering the
patients alone is not sufficient since it simply creates a need
for a special unit which relates patients to numbers. By incorporating that feature into the computer system and by also
including Soundex retrieval of records (so that a patient may
be identified at admission by name and supplementary
identifiers) we have made it possible to start the processing
on a timely basis.

One of the key uses of a data bank is to condense information and put all relevant information into a single source.
This means that there can only be one record per patient
regardless of the number of visits or admissions of the patient.
It is, of course, often desirable to indicate that multiple
admissions or visits have occurred, but this is secondary to
the goal of maintaining the use of a single record.

The combination of Soundex Retrieval with the computer-
based admissions system led to an active identification record
for each patient, which was accurate and ready to be used as
a basis for other information. This system was combined
with the on-line census entry for patient location within the
hospital. The Soundex file and history file became the first
modules in the Los Angeles County hospital information
system. With these factors as the first modules, the
development of other modular systems was anticipated.

D. Identification of Exceptions

In designing this system, account had to be taken of
the inevitable exceptions. With the cooperation of the hospital

registrar, we identified virtually all of the exception areas,
such as patients who are rushed through as a medical
emergency, patients who are police cases and are unwilling
to give their name, and patients who are children and unable
to identify themselves. The technique used in the Los Angeles
County system is the creation of records labeled John or Jane
Doe with numbers 1 through 999 which can be used to hold
treatment data on the patient until some verification of their
identity is accomplished. This method was merely an
adaptation of what the Registrar had been doing previously,
before a computer was considered.

E. Levels of Backup

If the hospital becomes dependent on the central system,
any systems failure becomes a major disaster. For this
reason multiple levels of backup are required. The standard
techniques of using duplicate tapes, disks, etc., were, of
course, available. In addition, the on-line system has a
logging file, and there is a security backup plus an entirely
separate system for updating with a logging file so that
current access to data is possible even if the primary system
fails. Then, just in case, we set up a system for providing
hard-copy backup and daily update, which to date has not been
used.

5

Hospital Information System Effectiveness

E. Jack Bond
Marketing Representative
McDonnell Automation Co.
St. Louis, Missouri

PREFACE

One of the most vexing problems associated with the
introduction of information systems to a hospital is the
measurement of its effectiveness. Generally, one would
expect the system to reduce the cost of health care and to
improve its quality, or both. Unfortunately, some of these
benefits are intangible and hard to assess. It is possible
(though not necessarily easy) to determine whether the average
cost of the admitting service per patient has decreased or
increased. Improved reporting, faster access to clinical
laboratory reports or a reduced number of errors in patient
files (which all contribute to an improvement in the quality of
patient care), however, are difficult to quantify. To these
considerations must be added the fact that an automated system
cannot be simply overlaid on a manual system if it is to be
effective. Rather, systems must be redesigned and personnel
redistributed.

For these reasons, there have been relatively few
carefully documented studies of the cost effectiveness of
hospital information systems. This chapter presents one such
attempt. Several hypotheses regarding the effectiveness of a
shared hospital information system are stated and results are
presented. The chapter represents a first step in the direction of quantifying the evaluation process.

I. INTRODUCTION

In 1960 the Sisters of the Third Order of St. Francis
(OSF), Peoria, Illinois, established a data processing center
which would eventually centralize all of the data handling
requirements of this organization. Unit record equipment
was used in establishing the system to be replaced in 1963
with computer equipment [1].

II. CENTRAL DATA BASE

In 1965, exhaustive studies indicated the need to
communicate the information requirements via telecommunications to a central data base. The concept of sharing centralized equipment was reconfirmed as the most economical
method to accomplish this goal. In addition to the economics
involved, it also allowed OSF hospitals the use of sophisticated
equipment and staff which would otherwise not be available to
them on an individual basis. The conclusions of this study
indicated a two-phase approach to installation of the systems
requirements of OSF by 1970.

1. Phase 1 involved the development of an on-line
    network which would control all administrative and
    accounting data of OSF.

2. Phase II involved an on-line, real-time shared
    hospital information system (SHIS) which dealt with
    data concerning patients during their stay in OSF
    hospitals. The objective of this system was to
    automate clerical information data-handling which
    would directly effect the quality of delivering health
    care within OSF hospitals, thus, freeing valuable
    skilled nursing personnel with time to provide more
    meaningful care to hospitalized patients.

A. Results of Phase I

Phase I was cost-justified. Design of the system and
eventual implementation was funded by OSF. Complete installation on-line was achieved in 1967.

B. Phase II

Phase II was not cost-justified and more appropriately
fell into the category of operations research and development.
OSF was incapable of funding the development costs associated
with this system when related to the risk of success. Therefore, outside funds were sought and eventually obtained through
Public Health Service Research Grant Number HM00504,
Division of Hospital and Medical Facilities. Later the project
was reassigned to the Health Care Technology Program,

National Center for Health Services Research and Development,
Department of Health, Education, and Welfare under Grant
Number HS00083-03.   The initial grant request envisioned a
4. 5 million dollar project involving the OSF's eleven (11)
hospitals covering a five (5) year period of time.   Later the
project was scaled down to a pilot demonstration of three (3)
hospitals and approximately 1. 5 million dollars over a three
(3) year period.   The hospitals involved were selected for
their diverse environment, i. e. , a large teaching hospital, a
small rural hospital, and a medium-sized modern urban
hospital.   The project was cut back to include admitting,
radiology, and laboratory as the first applications, with the
other ancillary service departments to follow.

C.   System Characteristics

During the initial phases of the project, it became
evident that physicians would not use the terminals to enter
doctors' orders.   Since the system was to be used in an actual
working environment affecting the total hospital operation, we
selected a user-oriented terminal (the IBM 1050/92 matrix
keyboard).   Video display units were selected for use in
admitting and radiology.   We proceeded on the basis that when
and if physicians eventually were to use the terminals, the
network would be in place and the system would be upgraded
to handle this change in operating philosophy.

1.   Software and Hardware Configuration

We had planned on using the IBM Corporation's Medical
Information System Program (MISP).   These plans were later

abandoned due to certain software problems [2]. As a result
of this decision, we designed and implemented our own
executive which operates under IBM's OS utilizing QTAM.
Equipment at the data center was configured and installed as
follows:

IBM 360	2050, 512K CPU
	2314 Disk Facility
	2401 (4) Tape Drives
	2540 Card Reader
	1403 Printer
	2701 CRT Transmission
	2703 Transmission Control
	2711 (2) Line Adapters

The hospital equipment was configured and installed
as follows:

Peoria (St. Francis Hospital)

22	1050/52/92 Nurses Stations
2	1050/52/53/92/93 Laboratory
1	1050/52/53 Laboratory
1	1050/52/92/93 Radiology
1	1050/53 Radiology
1	1050/52 Admitting
2	1050/53/53 Admitting
5	2260 CRT Admitting
3	2260 CRT Radiology
1	2848 CRT Controller

Rockford (St. Anthony's Hospital)

9	1050/52/92 Nurses Stations
1	1050/52/53/92/93 Laboratory
1	1050/52/53 Laboratory
1	1050/52/53/92/93 Radiology
1	1050/53/53 Admitting
1	1050/52 Admitting
2	2260 CRT Radiology
2	2260 CRT Admitting
1	2848 CRT Controller
1	Mohawk Transceiver and Line Printer

Galesburg   (St. Mary's Hospital)

5	1050/52/92 Nurses Station
1	1050/52/53 Admitting
1	1050/52/53/92/93 Laboratory
1	1050/52/53/92/93 Radiology
1	2260 CRT Admitting
2	2260 CRT Radiology
1	2848 CRT Controller
1	Mohawk Transceiver and Line Printer

2. Communications Network

The following communications network was installed:

Peoria   (St. Francis Hospital)

30	Local Lines 150 BPS
1	High Speed Line 2400 BPS

Rockford   (St. Anthony's Hospital)

4	4 Channel Long Lines 150 BPS
1	High Speed Line 2400 BPS

Galesburg   (St. Mary's Hospital)

2	4 Channel Long Lines 150 BPS
1	High Speed Line 2400 BPS

3. Operational Costs

Operational cost of the foregoing, excluding staff, amounts to approximately $2.25 per occupied bed day. This includes the applications of admitting, radiology, and laboratory. The centralized computer equipment, as shown above, should be able to handle the remainder of the ancillary service departments of the hospital. The completed system envisions a data base of all physician orders throughout the hospital.

III. RESULTS OF STUDY

A. First Hypothesis Tested

1. Hypothesis A - Patient Nursing Care

Implementation of SHIS will increase patient care through increased nurse utilization by patient category. (Patient care is defined as the sum of the time spent in patient-nursing personnel interaction.)

The experimental model produced five dependent variables which were measured to evaluate this hypothesis.

    a. Care hours performed per hour per patient

    b. Care coverage by skill level

    c. Demand coverage by skill level

    d. Productivity

    e. Clock hours per patient day

One of the objectives of SHIS was to get the nurse away from the desk and back to the patient. This was to accomplished by transferring the clerical demands from the nurse to the computer system. Relief from non care activities would allow better organization and, therefore, result in better matching of work with skill requirements. The increase in available time would also allow the amount of care to be matched to the care requirements of the patients. The evaluation of Hypothesis A will indicate the degree to which implementation of SHIS contributed.

2. Conclusions

    a. In ten of twenty cases, the data from the measured variables supports the hypothesis. In seven cases

the data indicates that SHIS has had no effect; in
three cases the data was inconclusive.

b. Of particular importance is the effect that SHIS had
on clerical workload. Based on demand coverage
data for RN-LPN-TA staff, the implementation of
SHIS has eliminated or reorganized clerical activities equal to the following percentages of the total
nursing time:

    (1) Post Partum: Peoria   (4%)
    (2) 3A: Peoria   (2%)
    (3) Urology: Peoria   (8%)
    (4) 400S: Galesburg   (no effect)

c. The data indicated many significant improvements
in the admissions procedures:

    (1) Significantly less time is required to admit a
        patient under SHIS.
    (2) SHIS has provided activity displacement of over
        19% of the productive work requirements of the
        department.
    (3) SHIS has significantly improved staff utilization
        and has smoothed the workload through activity
        reorganization and through patient throughput
        time reductions from 20% to 55%.

B.   Second Hypothesis Tested

1. Hypothesis B – Quality of Patient Care

Implementation of SHIS will improve the quality of
patient-nursing care and the quality of communications which
affects patient care. (Quality of patient-nursing care is
defined as the relative amount of time spent by each skill

level - RN, LPN, AIDE, and CLERK - in administering patient care as compared to the hospital's goal.)

The experimental model produced two dependent variables which were measured to evaluate this hypothesis.

a. Care quality by activity skill goal

b. Quality of communications

One of the objectives of SHIS was to improve the over- all efficiency of the nursing staff by having the appropriate level of skill employee perform the appropriate tasks. This cost-effectiveness improvement was to be accomplished by better organization and effective application of the staff rather than changing the techniques of administering individual items of patient care. By relieving the higher skills of nonessential activities, the available time would allow more timely perfor- mance and a greater quantity of nurse-patient related activi- ties. The desirability of having the activity performed by the required skill is a measure of quality of patient care.

Information transfer is a necessary aspect of accurate diagnosis and performance of quality patient care. An objec- tive of SHIS was to reduce the clerical effort and improve the quality or accuracy of communication functions. For evalua- tion, an improvement in quality of communications and, indirectly, quality of patient care, would be recognized when the number of errors or defects were reduced. The evaluation of Hypothesis B will indicate the degree to which implementa- tion of SHIS contributed to this objective.

2. Conclusions

a. Quality of skill utilization may have been improved with the introduction of SHIS, but not significantly. This is primarily attributed to the fact that the hospitals have not yet adjusted their entire organization to the system.

b. Implementation of SHIS has significantly improved the quality of communications in every significant category that was affected by the system. The probability of erroneous information being introduced into the patient care process was reduced by more than 20% in those areas served by SHIS. Thus SHIS has made a significant contribution to improved patient care accuracy.

C.   Third Hypothesis Tested

1. Hypothesis C – Response Times

Implementation of SHIS will improve timeliness. (Timeliness is defined as the elapsed time from issuance to consummation of a patient service demand.)

The experimental model produced ten dependent variables which were measured to evaluate this hypothesis.

a. Time to admit preadmitted patient

b. Time to admit walk-in patient

c. Time to respond to call light

d. Time from physician's written order to requisition

e. Time from order entry to receipt in ancillary desk

f. Time from ancillary desk to start of process

g. Time from test completion to availability at
ancillary desk

h. Time from result availability to nursing station

i. Time from result receipt in nursing to chart

j. Time waiting for service in radiology department

One of the objectives of SHIS was to improve the efficiency of the hospital staff and the quality of patient care by reducing the waiting or reaction time when services or action is required. The evaluation of Hypothesis C will indicate the degree to which implementation of SHIS contributed to this objective.

2. Conclusions

a. In the Peoria nursing stations overall improvement
to order flow in excess of 44% was created by SHIS.

b. In the Galesburg nursing station overall improvement to order flow in excess of 36% was created by
SHIS.

c. In the Peoria laboratory overall improvement to
order flow in excess of 34% was created by SHIS.

d. In the Galesburg laboratory overall improvement
to order flow in excess of 21% was created by SHIS.

e. In the Peoria radiology department, the introduction
of SHIS reduced the overall indirect patient care
processing time by 27%.

    f.   In the Galesburg radiology department, the overall indirect patient care processing time decreased by more than 25%.

    g.   In the admissions department no response time improvement occurred as a result of reduced productivity due to the improved efficiency of SHIS.

    h.   The introduction of SHIS has been matched by a 25% drop in verbal communications relating to patient service demands.

D. Fourth Hypothesis Tested

1. Hypothesis D – Transportation and Scheduling

Implementation of SHIS is to be the foundation for a dynamic transportation and work scheduling system.

Since a qualitative evaluating of this hypothesis was to be made, no data was measured using the experimental model. However, hospital operations during the experimental periods were observed to obtain information for evaluating this hypothesis.

At the beginning of the experimental demonstration, it was noted that the installation of SHIS might provide the necessary tools of communications and a data base for a dynamic transportation and work scheduling system. The evaluation of Hypothesis D will indicate the degree to which implementation of SHIS contributed to this objective.

2. Observations

a. SHIS has given the laboratory department the data base for scheduling sample collections and work flow.

b. SHIS has given the radiology department a more complete data base for scheduling of patients, technicians, and transportation personnel.

c. Through the admissions subsystems for patient census, discharges and transfers, SHIS has embodied substantially all of the information required to plan better nursing staff assignments based on patient census and actual patient needs.

d. Evidence of a reduction of transfers in excess of 10% on the experimental floors has indicated that SHIS has provided better organization of room availability information for the initial assignment of patients to rooms.

e. When other ancillary service departments are tied into the system it will be possible for SHIS to assist with the elimination of scheduling conflicts for patients, personnel and facilities.

3. Conclusions

It is apparent that SHIS is a useful tool for transportation coordination and patient care scheduling for the hospitals who are prepared to exploit it to the fullest extent.

E.   Fifth Hypothesis Tested

1. Hypothesis E - Cost of Patient Services

Implementation of SHIS utilizing a shared data center will be achieved without significantly affecting the cost of patient services.

The experimental model produced three dependent variables which were measured to evaluate this hypothesis.

a. Productivity

b. Cost of routine patient services

c. Cost of laboratory and radiology services by individual procedures

The objectives of the preceding hypotheses were to improve the quantity and quality of patient care. Underlying each hypothesis was the objective that the improvements would be achieved without increasing the cost to the patient by off-setting the system operating costs with reductions in labor costs at both the nursing stations and in the ancillary departments. The evaluation of Hypothesis E will indicate the degree to which implementation of SHIS contributed to these objectives.

2. Conclusion

Data from the experimental model indicates that activities equivalent to $0.46/patient day at St. Francis and $1.28/patient day at St. Mary's have been displaced by SHIS. These savings were primarily generated by the reduction of clerical activities of RN's and LPN's ($0.21 for Peoria and $1.02 for Galesburg), less processing time in the admitting office

($0. 12 for Peoria, same estimated for Galesburg), and improved efficiency in the radiology department at Peoria ($0. 13) and laboratory department at Galesburg ($0. 14).

Observations indicate that these savings have only been realized in the Peoria radiology and Galesburg laboratory; the nursing staffs and admitting office staffs have not been reduced. The Peoria laboratory and Galesburg radiology yielded no savings because they have not yet adapted their operations to SHIS.

Analysis indicates that additional savings of $1. 00/ patient day at St. Francis and $1. 75/patient day at St. Mary's could be realized if the system's capabilities were fully utilized. Potential savings from patient routine services are estimated at $0. 55 per patient day for Peoria and $1. 30 for Galesburg. The admitting office would provide $0. 10, the radiology departments $0. 15 and the laboratories $0. 20/ patient day. This analysis does not project the potential savings from application of the system in other areas, nor does it include the extra revenue that may result from reducing "lost" charges.

It should be noted that potential cost savings of the SHIS cannot be realized until the hospital staff is completely integrated with the computer system. The relative savings versus operating costs could not be evaluated because development is a primary cost of the present system.

IV. CONCLUSIONS FOR PHASE II

At St. Francis Hospital, Peoria, the overall effect
upon physicians was clearly favorable. In the laboratory, the
format was considered an improvement, however, there was
dissatisfaction expressed in the organization of laboratory
data in the chart. The laboratory interim report improved
timeliness of reporting considerably. The interim x-ray
report was the most popular application received by the
doctors. The physicians at this hospital showed a strong
positive attitude concerning the application of future computer
technology to the handling of hospital data. In general, the
physicians were pleased with the results of the system at
St. Francis Hospital.

Physicians at St. Anthony's Hospital, Rockford,
expressed a clearly unfavorable opinion of SHIS. As a matter
of fact, no physician felt the SHIS program had improved his
overall satisfaction with hospital practice. In the laboratory,
most physicians felt the interim report had no effect on timeliness of reporting. These physicians, like St. Francis, felt
that the organization of laboratory data in the chart had not
been significantly improved. A majority of the physicians
felt that the x-ray interim report was helpful; however, they
were critical of the tendency of radiologists to include less
detail in the final report. Many of the physicians expressed a
positive attitude in the use of the computer systems in hospitals.

Physicians at St. Mary's Hospital, Galesburg, were
approximately evenly divided as to a favorable opinion concer-

ning SHIS. It is interesting to note that the general response
of physicians fell between the clearly favorable opinion at
St. Francis and the distinctly unfavorable reply from
St. Anthony's. Here, again, the laboratory system had the
strongest negative influence upon the ultimate acceptance of
the total system. Counterbalancing this poor opinion of the
laboratory was a strong positive response in favor of the
radiology system. Once again, as at the other hospitals, the
most popular descriptor of physicians' attitudes about the
future of SHIS was "positive".

An analysis of the combined responses of the physicians revealed a slightly favorable opinion of the system.
Votes were clearly in favor of retaining the system; support
for the radiology application overcame the cool reception
given to the laboratory system. However, in October, 1970,
the laboratory results reporting summary sheet was reorganized and displayed in a fashion which was most favorable to
the practicing physicians at all three hospitals.

ACKNOWLEDGMENT

This investigation was supported by a research grant
from the Health Care Technology Program, National Center
for Health Services Research and Development, Department
of Health, Education, and Welfare under Grant Number
HS00083-03.

REFERENCES

1. Walter S. Huff, Jr., "Shared Computer Time: Big
    Benefits for Small Hospitals," Modern Hospital,
    November 1969.

2. Progress Report, 1968, Shared Hospital Information
    System, The Sisters of the Third Order of St. Francis,
    General Office, Peoria, Illinois.

3. Progress Report, 1967, Shared Hospital Information
    System, The Sisters of the Third Order of St. Francis,
    Central Administrative Office, Peoria, Illinois.

4. Experimental Model – Demonstration of a Shared Hospital
    Information System, June 13, 1968, The Sisters of the
    Third Order of St. Francis, Central Administrative
    Office, Management Services Division, Peoria, Illinois.

5. Findings of Pre-Installation Control Period, August 1,
    1969, Demonstration of a Shared Hospital Information
    System (Including Appendix), The Sisters of the Third
    Order of St. Francis, General Office, Management
    Services Division, Peoria, Illinois.

6. Walter S. Huff, Jr., Et Al, "Knowing and Controlling
    Costs in a Hospital," Journal of Hospital Financial
    Management Association, May 1969.

6

Data Processing Techniques for Multitest Screening and Hospital Facilities *

Morris F. Collen
Director Medical Methods Research
Permanente Medical Group, Oakland, California

I. INTRODUCTION

Multitest laboratories with automated, electronic, and computer equipment used for routine periodic health examinations have been described previously [1, 5], and an analysis of 39, 524 patients examined in 1 year has been reviewed [2]. In December 1966, the laboratory in the Kaiser Foundation Hospital in Oakland, California, was enlarged and revised. The resulting greater usefulness and flexibility permitted examinations of men and women arriving in any order and allowed the laboratory to serve the medical center with regard to hospital admissions and preoperative evaluations.

---

* Reprinted by permission of Journal of Occupational Medicine from an article entitled "The Multitest Laboratory in Health Care," July 1969, Vol. 11, No. 7, by Morris F. Collen, M. D., and Lou F. Davis, M. A. ; and by permission of the Proceedings of the IEEE from an article entitled "A Pilot Data System for a Medical Center," November 1969, Vol. 57, No. 11, by E. E. Van Brunt, M. F. Collen, L. S. Davis, E. Besag, and S. J. Singer.

An automated multitest laboratory can significantly
affect the efficiency and economy of the delivery of health
services by a medical center to its patients and community.
Such a laboratory can operate most effectively when associated
with a medical center comprising inpatient and outpatient
services; it can then function as an automated multipurpose
laboratory providing screening and diagnostic services, immu-
nization, and health evaluation to both hospital and office
patient.

In the future it is likely that larger hospitals in every
community of 100,000 or more will be affiliated with an automated multitest laboratory, which will conduct admission and
preoperative examinations for hospital patients, and which
will be utilized by office patients for periodic health examinations, health evaluations for special purposes (industrial,
insurance, etc.), early sickness consultations, and diagnostic
surveys. These multitest laboratories undoubtedly will be
affiliated with a regional computer center which will provide
data processing services through connecting telephone lines.
Automated multitest laboratories will provide more data on
more people, and more data on each individual, more accurately and at a lower unit cost than is now possible.

II.   TESTING PROCEDURES

This laboratory processes 2000 cases monthly. A
patient proceeds from Station 1 to Station 20 in a period of two
to three hours (see Figs. 1 to 11). During this time, he
receives the following tests and procedures.

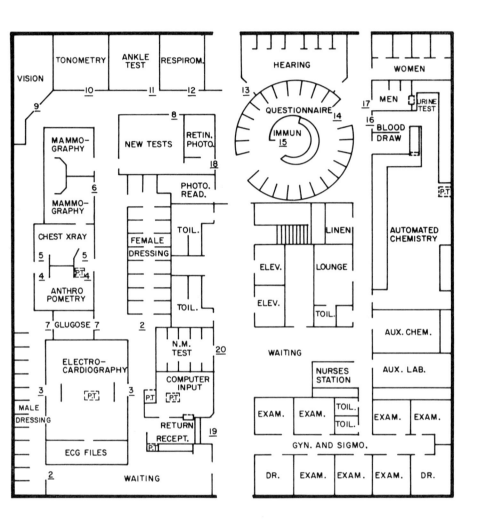

Fig. 1. Multitest laboratory lay-out.

A. Test Stations

Station 1. Patients register at the desk approximately every three minutes. Here they receive a clipboard containing

a medical questionnaire form and a deck of cards (prepunched
for computer input with their medical record number) on
which are to be recorded the test results at each station. The
patient's electrocardiogram card is dispatched by pneumatic
tube from the reception desk to Station 3, so the technician
there is informed of patient sequence.

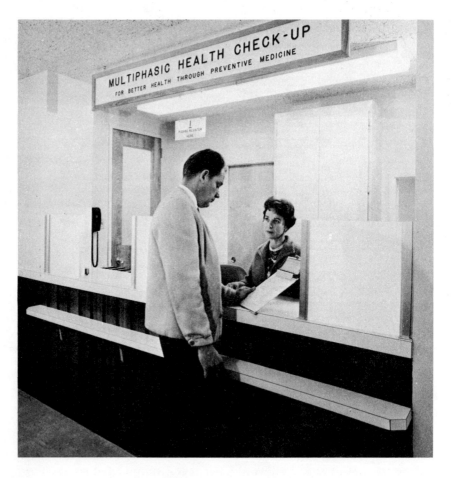

Fig. 2. Station 1: Reception desk.

Station 2. The patient removes the upper body garments in a dressing booth and puts on a disposable paper gown.

Station 3. Six electrocardiogram (ECG) leads (AVR, AVL, AVF, V_1, V_3, V_5) are simultaneously recorded by means of a direct optical recording oscillograph. The ECG's are subsequently read by a cardiologist who records his interpretations on a "mark-sense" card, using pencil marks that can be sensed directly by a card-reading machine for input to the computer.

Station 4. Weight and skinfold thickness: the subscapular and triceps are measured with a caliper; and the data are key punched into the patient's anthropometry test card. By means of an automated anthropometer, height and transverse body measurements are recorded directly into the patient's punched card within 3 minutes.

Station 5. A 70 mm posterioanterior chest roentgenogram is obtained, to be read subsequently by a radiologist who records his interpretations on a mark-sense punch card.

Station 6. Mammography is performed on all women aged 48 and over. Cephalocaudal and lateral views of each breast are taken. Mammograms are subsequently read by a radiologist who records his interpretations on a mark-sense card. The patient then returns to the booth in Station 2 and redresses.

Station 7. The patient ingests 75 g of glucose solution in 240 ml of cold, carbonated water dispensed from a vending machine. The time of glucose ingestion is recorded by an automatic time stamp on the back of the card, and the patient is assigned a sequencing number from 1 to 24 for control purposes and for later assignment to a booth in Station 14.

Station 8. Supine pulse rate and blood pressure are measured by an automated instrument and directly punched into a card.

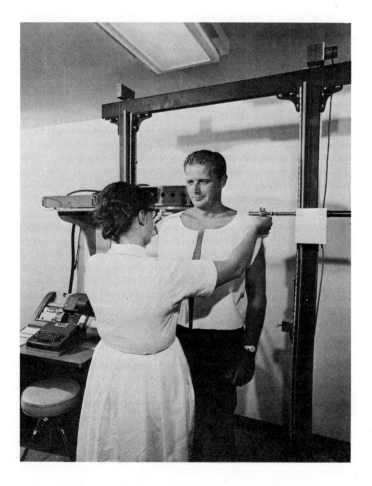

Fig. 3. Station 4: Weight and skinfold.

Station 9. Visual acuity is tested by reading a wall chart, and the results are recorded on a mark-sense card.

Station 10. Ocular tension is measured by a tonometer, and the reading recorded on a mark-sense card.

Station 11. The Achilles reflex one-half relaxation time is measured to screen for hypothyroidism.

Station 12. A 1-second, 2-second, and total forced expiratory vital capacity and peak flow is measured with a spirometer and directly punched into a card.

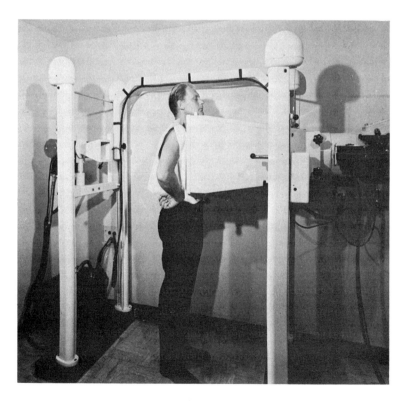

Fig. 4. Station 5: Chest x-ray.

Station 13. Hearing is tested with an automated audio-meter for six frequencies in each ear, and the graphed readings transferred to a mark-sense card.

Station 14. The self-administered medical question-naire form which the patient received at Station 1, and which has been completed during any waiting periods between stations, is now audited by a nurse. The patient is then assigned to one of 24 questionnaire booths in accordance with the sequencing number received at Station 7. In this booth, the patient

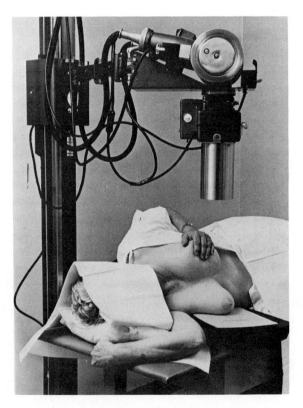

Fig. 5. Station 6: Mammography.

receives a letter box containing a deck of 207 prepunched
cards, each having a single dichotomous question printed on
the card.   Typical "inventory by systems" questions have been
selected that are judged to be medically of value in discrimi-
nating patients with specific diseases from those nondiseased
[3].   The patient responds to each question by taking the card
from the top section of the divided letter box and dropping the
card into the middle section if his answer to the question is
"yes," or into the bottom section if his answer is "no."   This

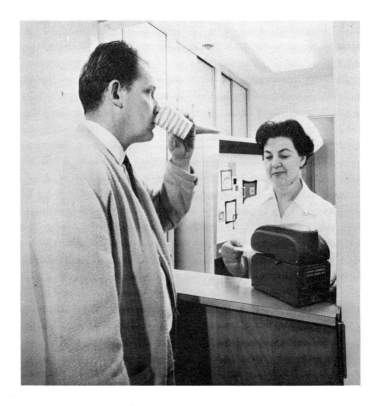

Fig. 6. Station 7: Glucose.

procedure automatically sorts "yes" responses for direct
input to the computer by means of a card-reading machine.

In order to test-retest the "yes" responses when the
patient has completed sorting all the questions, the nurse
removes the "yes" cards from the middle section of the box,
places them back in the upper section and asks the patient to
go through them once more "to be sure the answers are yes."
This additional step decreases the "false" yes responses by
about 10%.

Station 15. As a part of the preventive medical
program, the patient may here receive a booster dose of
tetanus toxoid, using a high-pressure jet injector.

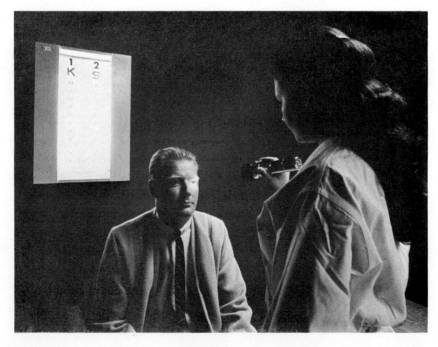

Fig. 7. Station 9: Visual acuity.

Station 16. When an hour has elapsed since ingestion of the glucose challenge dose, the patient is called from his assigned questionnaire booth and is sent to the laboratory where blood samples are drawn for a hemoglobin test, white blood cell count, venereal disease research laboratories test for syphilis (VDRL), and blood grouping. The test values are

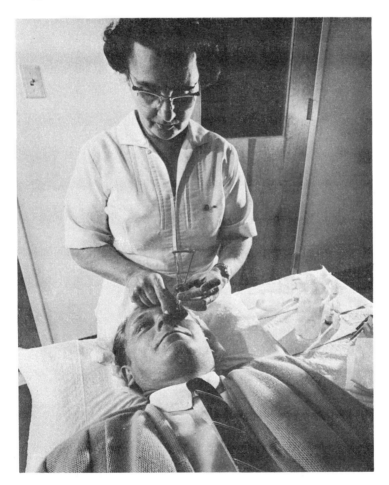

Fig. 8. Station 10: Ocular tension.

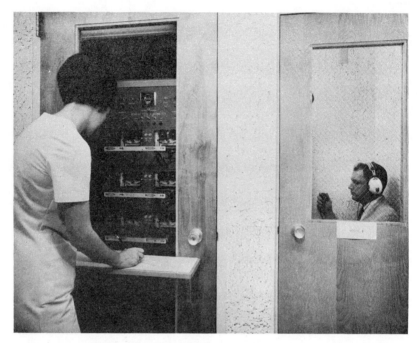

Fig. 9. Station 13: Hearing test.

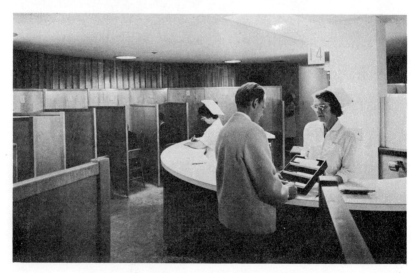

Fig. 10. Station 14: Medical questionnaire.

recorded on mark-sense cards. From a single 2-ml sample of serum, at least 8 blood chemistry determinations (serum glucose, creatine, albumin, total protein, cholesterol, uric acid, calcium, and transaminase) are simultaneously done by an automated chemical analyzer; test results are directly punched into cards.

Station 17. A urine specimen is collected, and tests are done for bacteriuria (cultured 6 hours with triphenyltetrazolium chloride), and for pH, blood, glucose, and protein

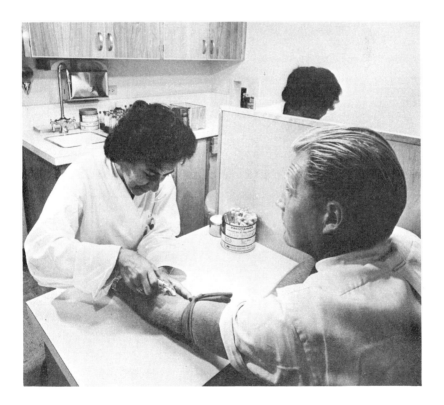

Fig. 11. Station 16: Blood sample.

(paper strip tests).   The results are entered on the patient's
test card.

Station 18.   The patient returns to his questionnaire
booth.   When he has completed the questionnaire, he proceeds
to Station 19.

Station 19.   The patient returns to the registration
area and gives the receptionist the clipboard containing the
marked and punched cards and the questionnaire form.   He
now receives a second box of questionnaire cards, for psychological testing.

Station 20.   The patient again sits in a booth in this
station, and sorts 155 psychological questions into "true" and
"false" responses, using a sort box in the same manner he
did with the medical questionnaire in Station 14.

By the time the patient has completed the psychological
questionnaire, the "on-line" computer processing has been
completed, and supplemental tests and appointments, "advised"
by the programmed rules of the computer, are arranged for
the patient.

Routinely advised are a sigmoidoscopy for all patients
aged 40 or more and, for women, a gynecologic examination
with cervical smear for cancer detection.

B.   Data Processing Requirements for Test Stations

Most of the data generated in the automated multitest
laboratory is recorded on prepunched or mark-sense cards to
permit its immediate introduction into the data processing

system. As an "on-line" procedure, while the patient is in
Station 20, the computer processes the information from (1)
the punched cards from blood pressure, spirometry, anthropometry and chemistry; (2) the prepunched sorted cards from
the medical questionnaire box; and (3) the reproduced mark-
sense cards from hearing, vision, and urine paper strip tests,
hemoglobin determination, and white cell count. The punched
cards are read into a data communication system, and the
data transmitted via telephone line to the central computer in
a separate building.

The computer processor goes through a program
routine containing various test limits and decision rules, and
prints out a report (see Table I) constituting "advice" as to
any additional procedures that should be done before the next
visit and the time and length of the follow-up appointment with
the physician. These "advice" rules have been established
previously by the internists. For example, if the 1-hour
serum glucose is greater than a predetermined "normal" limit
for the patient's age and the hours since last food ingestion,
the computer prints out instructions to the receptionist to
return the patient to Station 16 to draw blood for a 2-hour
serum glucose. If a serious abnormality is detected, an
earlier appointment with the physician is advised.

As an "off-line" procedure, the computer collates and
stores the remaining information on the random access disk
pack, which arrives a few days later (mark-sense card physician interpretations from the ECG and roentgenograms; the
remaining laboratory test reports; and the key-punched
medical questionnaire form). When all information has been

164 M. F. COLLEN

Table I. Example of a Computer-Generated Report.

PERMANENTE MEDICAL GROUP - OAKLAND
FINAL SUMMARY REPORT - MULTIPHASIC HEALTH CHECKUP - 2/07/67

```
DOE, JANE                                        DR. SMITH J J
M.R.NO. 9876543    BIRTHDATE 05-29  FEMALE       OAKL

  ANTHROPOMETRY: 127.5 LB.,   64.5 IN
**ECG: LT.VENT.HYPERTROPHY
**PHONOCARD: SYSTOLIC BASAL MURMUR
**SUPINE BLOOD PRESSURE: 165/80          SUPINE RADIAL PULSE:  76.

  RESPIROMETRY:        (NORMAL)                        (NORMAL)
  FEV 1 SEC:  1.9L  (OVER  1.2)     TOT. FVC:  2.5L  (OVER  2.1)
  FEV 2 SEC:  2.2L  (OVER      )    PEAK FLOW: 3.4L/S (OVER     )
**CHEST XRAY: CARDIAC ENLARGEMENT HEART/CHEST RATIO .51
  BREAST XRAY: NSA

  VISUAL ACUITY: R.E.20/40 OR BETTER      L.E.20/40 OR BETTER
  PUPILLARY ESCAPE: NO PUPILLARY ESCAPE
  OCULAR TENSION: R.E. NORMAL            L.E. NORMAL
**RETINAL PHOTO: MINIMAL DIABETIC RETINOPATHY
  HEARING: NO CLINICALLY SIGNIF.HEARING DEFECT
  PAIN RESPONSE TEST: 21 (NORM.8-35)
  ACHILLES REFLEX: 310MS (HYPERTHYROID 300-: NORM.250-380: HYPOTHYROID 350+)

  URINE: PH 6 **GLUCOSE MED.  PROTEIN 0    BLOOD 0     BACILLI NEG.
      **CLINITEST 3+4+         **ACETONE +
  VDRL 0          BLOOD GROUP AB      LATEX AGGLUT. 0
  HEMOGLOBIN 12.3 GM (NORM.12.0-14.5)  WHITE COUNT  9,000(NORM.4000-12,000
  SERUM:              (NORMAL)         SERUM:              (NORMAL)
**GLUCOSE (1 HR.) 310   MG (UNDER 245)  CHOLESTEROL 195   MG (140-270)
**GLUCOSE (2 HR.) 170   MG (UNDER 151)
  TOTAL PROT.    6.7 GM (5.8-7.9)      CALCIUM      9.5 MG (8.6-10.8)
  ALBUMIN        4.0 GM (3.0-5.0)      URIC ACID    3.9 MG (2.3-6.3)
  CREATININE     .90 MG (UNDER 1.2)    SGOT         21  U (UNDER 40)
* 2 HR.BLOOD DRAWN  10 MIN.LATE

**PATIENT RECEIVED THE FOLLOWING (ADVICE RULE) DIRECTIONS:
  901-REFER TO MEDICAL DROP-IN CLINIC STAT BECAUSE
      URINE SUGAR 3+4+ AND ACETONE +
  700-2 HR.BLOOD SUGAR

**CONSIDER REFER TO ASYMPT. DIABETES STUDY IF FOLLOW-UP CONFIRMS DIABETES.

PATIENT ANSWERED YES TO THESE QUESTIONS ON 1966 FORM:
  249-HAD BAD REACTION OR SENSITIVITY TO PENICILLIN?
IN THE PAST MONTH:
  434-THROAT BEEN SORE ALMOST EVERY DAY?
IN THE PAST 6 MONTHS:
  450-SHORTNESS OF BREATH WITH USUAL WORK OR ACTIVITY?
IN THE PAST YEAR:
  476-REPEAT PAIN,PRESSURE,TIGHT FEELING IN CHEST IN MIDDLE OF BREAST BONE?
  478-REPEAT PAIN,PRESSURE,TIGHT FEELING IN CHEST WHEN SITTING STILL?
  482-REPEATED PAIN OR PRESSURE, IN CHEST WHEN WALK FAST,LEFT ON REST?
  483-REPEATED PAIN,PRESSURE OR TIGHT FEELING IN CHEST FORCED STOP WALKING?
  484-REPEATED PAIN OR PRESSURE, IN CHEST LASTING MORE THAN 10 MINUTES?
  574-ALWAYS HAVE TO GET UP FROM SLEEP TO URINATE?

** CONSIDER ABNORMAL,OR POSSIBLE VARIATION FROM NORMAL
NSA=NO SIGNIFICANT ABNORMALITY
* NOTE
```

received and stored, the computer produces a printed summary
of all test reports and questions answered "yes."

At the time of the patient's first office visit, the internist reviews the summary report and directs further history
toward elaborating the questions to which the patient has
answered "yes," and to the test abnormalities reported from
the automated multitest laboratory (see Fig. 12). He completes

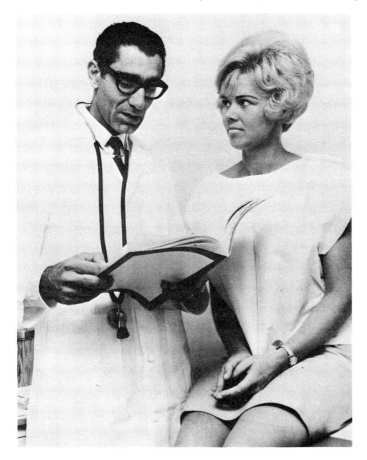

Fig. 12. Internist directs further history taking.

his physical examination, records the findings and diagnoses
on a preprinted form, which can be automatically scanned by
an optical mark reader or entered by electric typewriter
directly into the patient's computer medical record. He then
arranges whatever medical care is necessary for his patient
in the usual way.

III. HOSPITAL-BASED REAL-TIME SYSTEM

A. Nonadministrative Applications

In general, the implementation of electronic data
processing (EDP) techniques in other than administrative
areas of hospital care has proved to be a difficult process [6].
There are many reasons for this, including the great inertia
of the traditional medical process and consequent apparent
resistance to change, difficulty in standardizing elements of
the medical process, the dynamic nature of medical research
and development and the consequent need for frequent change,
and the enormous cost in dollars and technical manpower
involved in attempting to adapt as yet rather inflexible EDP
techniques to such conditions. The difficulty is further
compounded by a lack of standardization in the computing and
allied industries, and the problems of interdisciplinary
communication.

If data input terminals are to be used successfully in
the hospital, it is necessary to integrate the planning for and
the implementation of the data system into each hospital
department's operations. Accordingly, all our planning and
decision making has been and will continue to be with the

support and concurrence of supervisory department personnel.
To further facilitate interdisciplinary communication and
maximize user acceptance, we train physicians, laboratory
technologists, nurses, etc., in necessary aspects of data
processing technology. In addition, education and training
programs for users have developed concurrently with the data
system itself.

For reasons stated above it is apparent that a multipurpose hospital data system must evolve in a modular fashion
in order to meet its long term objectives. Such objectives
should include certain general elements which may be vital to
survival of the system: (a) reliability and economy; (b) capability of sufficiently smooth integration into professional
activities so that user acceptance is assured; (c) operational
characteristics that permit evaluation of the system, both in
terms of its cost and its impact on hospital and professional
activities; (d) establishment of a data base which is compatible
not only with clinical service but also with various research
requirements; and (e) the capacity for progressive expansion
of the number and quality of services to the professional and
nonprofessional user.

Over the past several years, this facility has studied
numerous EDP applications in the course of developing an
automated multiphasic screening project. This project currently processes data on more than 40,000 outpatients each
year, and utilizes such techniques as off-line batch processing,
telecommunications, and on-line generation of "advice rules"
to the laboratory [7]. In the past 2 years, attention has been

directed to the design and development of a hospital-based, multiterminal, real-time system for the handling of selected types of medical data. The immediate objective is to establish a limited medical data base for the 125,000 Kaiser Foundation Health Plan members who use its San Francisco Hospital, in order that specific statistical, epidemiological, and evaluative studies can be conducted. In so doing, the impact of the medical data system on the delivery of health services will be evaluated.

B.   General System Concept

The overall system orientation is that of a central computer facility, designed for both on-line and off-line processing of large volumes of all categories of medical data, linked in telecommunication mode with the "peripheral" hospital system 17 miles away. Within the hospital will be a smaller processor with its local storage and input-output devices, designed for multicategorical data acquisition, message routing, and as yet limited output service functions.

IV.   CENTRAL SYSTEM

A.   Functional Aspects

Fundamental to the programming strategies that have developed within the central system is the concept of a single repository for any and all data relating to an individual patient. A "patient computer medical record" (PCMR) has therefore been developed. The PCMR is a variable-length, variable-format, tree-structured record composed essentially of two classes of data: that which pertains to the patient (identification, administrative, and medical data), and that which constitutes the structure of the record (the nodes and indices which are used in locating specific areas in a given PCMR). The medical data section is divided into chronologically ordered patient "computer-defined visits." These visits in turn are divided into "parts," each of which contains a categorically different set of medical data, viz., medical history, observations by physicians, test results, diagnoses, prognoses, etc. Parts may be subdivided into "levels" for purposes of preserving medically meaningful associations of data. A medical record index, headed by the patient's unique seven-digit medical record number, initiates the PCMR. Several indices within each record facilitate rapid location of visits within sections and parts within visits. Input data is stored in the appropriate section, visit, and part in its encoded form. A more detailed description of the PCMR has been published elsewhere [8].

The design of the central computer system is such that a general programming strategy was devised in order to satisfy the numerous input, output, and processing operations necessary to maintain and update the dynamic sets of data that constitute medical records. This system, called the "medical function control system" (MFCS), is composed of fundamental routines which permit such operations as direct-access storage and retrieval and the handling of remote terminal as well as more conventional input and output devices. Within the MFCS various medical applications have been defined as

"functions, " and the MFCS is designed to control and coordinate the processing of multiple functions. It thus becomes
possible to treat the various medical applications in a modular
fashion, adding new applications as the need arises. Five
general program areas are encompassed by the MFCS,
entitled (1) medical record manipulation routines, (2) encoding
and translation routines, (3) medical language routines,
(4) medical function routines, and (5) a medical function
control program. The MFCS with its various medical functions operates under the control of an IBM 360 "operating
system allowing multiprogramming with a variable number of
tasks" (OS/MVT). Some medical functions may need to have
their own data sets, e. g. , lists of patients, normal ranges of
tests values, etc. Occasionally, multiple functions will need
access to the same data sets while some functions will require
temporary subsets of patient data. An operating principle,
however, is that the PCMR always is expected to have the
most current patient information and consequently is updated
before other data sets. A program routine called UPDATER
is solely responsible for the posting of all data to the PCMR.
Variably formatted input data are changed to standard image
by a "medical input description language" (MIDL) program
module and the data are passed to UPDATER. By use of additional subroutines, UPDATER requests exclusive use of the
PCMR and processes the standardized image data, posting
them to the PCMR and releasing the PCMR. when finished,
for use by other reading programs. A detailed outline of these
and other functions required for the central computer operation
has been published elsewhere [8].

B. Equipment Configuration

An equipment configuration (see Fig. 13) has been developed which initially permits limited patient medical information from three medical centers in the San Francisco Bay Area to be stored in the central computer's direct-access devices. It has been designed to permit modular expansion in order to accommodate increasing volumes of medical information as other peripheral hospital data systems are added.

The central system is built around an IBM 360/50 computer which operates as an on-line device and uses a 1-million-byte "large core" storage unit (see Fig. 14). A second or "backup" IBM 360/50 computer is used for testing, "debugging," and various batch processing operations: in the case of failure of the first computer, it is available for on-line operation by means of two manual switching devices. Each computer has access to its own input-output units and files, four IBM 2401 tape drives, an IBM 1403 N1 printer, and an IBM 2540 card-read-punch. The telecommunications control units which handle all remote terminal devices are capable of being connected to either computer by means of an IBM 2911 channel switching unit. Both computers have access to an IBM 2314 disk drive. In addition, a third printer, a third card reader, and two IBM 2321 data cell drives are available to either machine through an IBM 2911 channel switching device. The online computer will normally have the direct access to the data cell drives.

Since the basic premise of the MFCS is that the PCMR is fundamental to the general programming system, an explicit

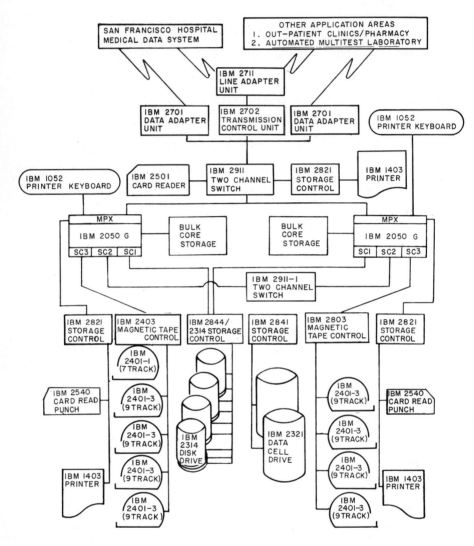

Fig. 13. Equipment configuration for a central computer system.

requirement of the MFCS is to have direct access to each patient's record. The PCMR data set will therefore reside in the two on-line data cells. As the size of this data set

increases with time, the MFCS can be adapted to handle
modular increases in the number of data cell drives. The
computer operating system (OS/MVT), MFCS, the transient
storage form of the PCMR (created for more efficient and
rapid manipulation following a request for a given record),
and other data sets, including an "English word dictionary"
and an "item catalogue," reside in the disk drives.

V. PERIPHERAL HOSPITAL SYSTEM

The peripheral site of operation is a 304-bed general
hospital providing acute medical care in essentially all medical
and surgical specialities. The hospital is available to about
125,000 members of the Kaiser Foundation Health Plan who

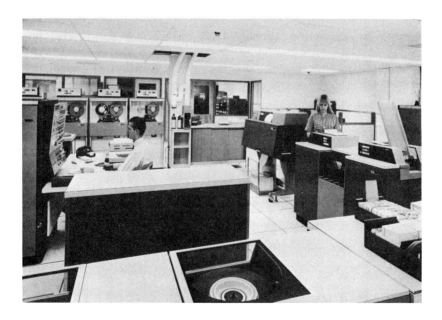

Fig. 14.   Central IBM 360/50 computer system.

reside in San Francisco.   The average occupancy is 85%.   The
average number of admissions to all services is 39 per day.

A.   Functional Requirements

The specific goals of the pilot data system are as
follows.

(a) To capture, on a continuous day-to-day basis, the
     medical data for each patient, in the following
     categories: (1) all diagnoses, (2) selected signs
     and symptoms, (3) results of all laboratory tests,
     (4) results of all x-ray, pathology, and EKG
     examinations, and (5) all drugs administered in the
     hospital.

(b) To transmit these data via telephone lines to the
     central computer system for storage in the PCMR.

(c) To provide limited service to the professional users
     in the form of several useful outputs, including
     printed (paper) and visually displayed (cathode ray
     tube) sets of data.

B.   Equipment Configuration

The basic hospital data processing equipment configuration includes the processor, limited random-access storage,
and over 50 input-output (I/O) devices from several manufacturing sources selected because they best fulfilled the functional
requirements outlined above.   The equipment configuration is
diagrammed in Figure 15.   Except for the IBM magnetic
tape selectric typewriter (MT/ST), all communications with
the central computer system are via telephone lines.   The two
Honeywell processors (DDP/516 and DDP/416) constitute the

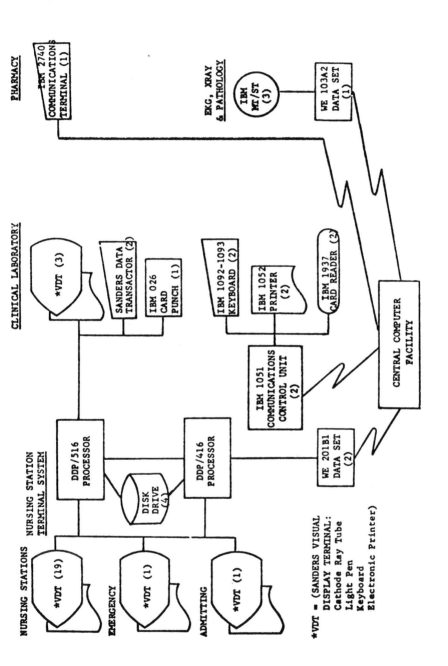

Fig. 15.   Equipment configuration for peripheral hospital system.

nucleus of the hospital data system. Potential core capacity
on each machine is 32K. The two computers access four data
disk F drives of 3, 136, 000 character total storage and 17
millisecond average access time. There exists the capacity
for four additional disk drives.

Computer programs are written in an interpretive
compiler language, file-oriented programming system (FOPS),
which has been supplied by Sanders Associates, Inc. All the
file design and applications systems that are described below –
the NSTS system, EKG, Surgical Pathology, etc. – are
programmed in this interpretive compiler language. This
JOSS-type language was developed to allow programmer and
medical personnel full advantage of light pen, keyboard, and
card-reader capabilities of the visual display terminals. Its
capabilities include (1) allowing programmers to write, enter,
and debug applications programs directly via the visual display
screen, and (2) numerous storage and retrieval operations
using a relatively small number of program statements. The
FOPS system consists of several monitor elements that control, under higher level application program direction, the
movement of data to and from the various hardware components,
including the disk files.

In this system the DDP/416 is necessary to compensate
for the difference in the high data-handling speed of the DDP/
516 and the comparatively low-speed operation of the electronic
printers, the 026 printing card punch, and the data phones.
This arrangement "liberates" the DDP/516 for higher speed
processing.

The Western Electric 201 B1 data sets transmit and receive binary data at a fixed rate over private telephone lines. The data set accepts asynchronous serial data from the DDP/416 interface and sends the data over the telephone lines at a transmission rate of 2400 bits per second. Each data set provides timing signals at the transmitting end. At the receiving end, bit synchronism is recovered and a timing lead is provided to the 360/50 computer interface. For the present application, the sets are wired to operate in a four-wire continuous operation mode with the transmitter always on. Two of these sets will be located at the hospital processor and paired sets are located in the central computer facility.

C. Reserve Power System

Since the hospital data system requires a backup power supply in case of electrical power failure, a noninterruptable ac power system was installed which contains four major components: (1) a constant voltage, current-limited battery charger; (2) storage batteries; (3) a static inverter; and (4) a diesel engine generator. During normal operation the ac line supplies power to the static battery charger, which in turn "float" charges the battery, and at the same time supplies dc power to the static converter. The inverter supplies ac power to the ac load. A synchronizing signal from the ac power lines maintains the phase and frequency of the inverter output the same as in the power line. The voltage regulator within the inverter maintains the ac load constant throughout the load range as well as periods of "equalizing" charge on the storage battery. Transient and steady-state power line

variations are isolated from the load by the regulating action
of the battery charger in conjunction with the filtering action
of the battery and the inverter.

If ac power failure occurs, the battery charger ceases
to operate; however, the battery continues to supply power to
the inverter in order to sustain the ac load without interrup-
tion. The inverter continues to operate on its own internal-
frequency reference, and is designed to maintain a constant
output voltage as battery voltage drops. Because of the limited
time the batteries can power the total hospital system, the
battery system is supplemented by the diesel engine generator.
Features of this element include automatic engine startup,
automatic switching of load to the generator without interrup-
tion, and transfer of load back to normal power when normal
ac supply is restored.

D. Nursing-Station Terminal System (NSTS)

This 21-terminal hospital data subsystem will be
distributed throughout the patient-care areas of the hospital.
It is that portion of the data system which will interface with
doctors and nurses and serve for data input and output for the
following classes of information: doctors' diagnoses, doctors'
orders (including drug and general nursing orders), confirmation of drug administration, and various test results (including
those from the clinical laboratory and x-ray departments). A
single nursing-station terminal is defined as a visual display
device with associated light-pen sensor, keyboard, card-
reader unit, and electronic printer.

The visual display device is a cathode ray tube (Sanders Associates model 708) with a 2048 character, vertically oriented matrix, arrayed in 40 lines of 51 characters each, in which may be displayed up to 1024 characters; the characters are stroke generated. The light-pen attachment is a hand held, photosensitive device of approximately fountain-pen size which, when positioned over a visible character on the cathode ray screen, activates a microswitch and generates an electric signal. The attached keyboard is a traditionally arranged cluster of 50 standard and 16 function keys, providing for 60 letters, numbers, and symbols and various editing capabilities. The attached card-reader unit contains two photoelectric assemblies. At the present time only one is in use and serves the function of decoding the user's punch-coded identification card. Thus a measure of control is achieved by providing that, before gaining access to the data stored in the computer, the operator must identify himself to the system.

The electronic printer is a modified Kleinschmidt model 311 used to provide a permanent record of that data that will be required for inclusion in the patient's chart. The printing rate is 40 characters per second. The printing noise has been reduced by greater than 85% by means of a silencing box which is designed to provide the operator with easy access to the printed copy as it emerges from the printer.

The NSTS is thus a computer-supported system of visual display terminals and printers designed to permit direct communication between hospital personnel and the computer for the purpose of entering into and extracting a variety of medical data from inpatient "computerized" medical records.

Data input may be accomplished at any nursing station
by an authorized user with a coded machine-readable identification card, who engages directly in a dialogue with the visual
display screen by means of either the light pen or the keyboard.
Data output may be in the form of a visual display or a permanent record produced by the printer. Such output methods
present legible and standardized information to the users.

Given sufficient computer support, an NSTS as
described is capable of being developed to embrace most types
of medical and administrative data input and output. The
primary applications of the present system, however, deal
only with those classes of information noted above.

The physician who places an order or records a diagnosis is responsible for the input of these data. Except in
unusual circumstances, the physician himself enters such data
directly. In the rare instance when this is manifestly impossible (when the physician is physically away from a terminal),
the data may be entered by specifically designated paramedical
personnel, but only upon the request of a physician. In any
case, the final responsibility for the validity of input data rests
with the person most capable of assuring its accuracy and
completeness. Thus, for purposes of verifying drug administration the appropriate nurse has the responsibility for data
input.

Activation of a visual display terminal by any person
is accomplished by insertion of his coded identification card
into the card-read station and depressing the function key
marked "signature." The processor searches its files to

verify the user's identification and functional classification,
and under program control establishes the paging sequences
to which he may have access. For the authorized user it
displays his name, the date, and the time. If he is not an
authorized user, an appropriate "error" message is displayed.
Under program control the inpatient census files are scanned
and the census local to the terminal in use is displayed. An
average local census is 25 patients with a range of from 5-33.

From this point on, by means of a series of rapid
light-pen selections, the user may identify any patient in the
hospital and page through a series of displays permitting input
of those classes of data outlined above. As appropriate selections are made, they are displayed in a so-called "verification"
area of the visual display screen until the user has completed
his task. A "terminal exit routine" has been established, such
that the final display exhibited is a summary of all data,
whether diagnostic, nursing orders, or drug administration,
which is destined for entry to the central computer PCMR or

for routing to a local hospital terminal for display or printing.
Thus, a final, rapid verification of data may be achieved by
the user prior to selection of a function item which results in
execution of the required printing and/or message routing
routines.

E. Clinical Laboratory System

In any general hospital the clinical laboratory plays a
vital role. Accordingly, results of all laboratory procedures
conducted on specimens from hospitalized patients are collected by several input methods, processed, reported to the
appropriate nursing stations, and stored in the appropriate
PCMR in the central computer facility.

The laboratory data processing subsystem consists of
the following equipment.

IBM 1050 data communications system which is a
multipurpose teleprocessing system used in a direct-inquire
and response (real-time) mode with the central computer
facility. Data is input to the 1050 system by manual keying
and punched-card methods. Output is in the form of a printed
document. The systems components are an IBM 1052 printer
keyboard, an IBM 1092/1093 programmed keyboard, a modified IBM 1001 (IBM 1937) data transmission terminal, and an
IBM 1051 control unit. Three such systems are used in the
laboratory.

IBM 026 printing card punch (modified by Sanders
Associates) is under control of the DDP/416 but can be
switched to manual control. It is used to punch cards for
purposes of test identification and reporting.

Three Sanders Associates visual display terminals with associated keyboard, light pen, card reader, and electronic printer will also be located in the clinical laboratory. They have the same characteristics as described in the previous section, and are similarly linked to the Honeywell DDP/615/416.

Table II indicates the distribution of the above equipment within the functional departments of the clinical laboratory.

Virtually all laboratory tests emanate directly from a physician's order (see Fig. 16). Immediately following selec-

TABLE II

Equipment Distribution Within the Clinical Laboratory

Laboratory department	Device
Specimen reception area	Visual display unit Data transactor Card punch Electronic printer
Hematology	Keyboard Printer Card Reader
Chemistry	Keyboard
Urine studies	Keyboard Printer Card reader
Serology – blood bank	Visual display unit Electronic printer
Bacteriology – parasitology	Visual display unit

tion of a laboratory test by the physician at a nursing-station terminal, and on recognition of the physician's order, the computer generates a laboratory test accession number and establishes a file containing patient and test identification data. This file is used for processing and retrieval after the test has been completed and is to be reported. The processor provides laboratory personnel with printed labels, distribution lists, "logs" of work ordered and in process, and, on demand, the verification of patient identification and validity of test result data. Additionally, "pickup" lists are provided to laboratory personnel for specimens to be collected in routine fashion, and test requisitions are produced at the nursing-station terminals for those tests for which specimens are to be collected by nursing or physician personnel.

Laboratory test reports entered into the data trans-actors[*] and cathode ray tube terminals[+] will be stored and queued in the hospital system and printed (see Fig. 17) at the appropriate nursing stations at intervals through the day. The

---

[*] Digital laboratory data is entered via the transactor as follows. (a) The patient is identified by inserting a Hollerith-coded punched card into the card-read slot on the transactor. (b) The test is identified by slewing to the appropriate English word block on the scroll. (c) The digital test result is entered via the keyboard. (d) The entire set of data is dispatched by depressing a "send" key.

[+] Both digital and English word laboratory data are entered via the cathode ray tube visual display terminal. The terminal is activated and the technologist identified by use of the card-reader function. Appropriate keyboard and light-pen selections identify the patient, test name, and other identifiers as required. The entire set of data is dispatched by light-pen selection of a print or finish function.

```
                                           DAY   113
PATIENT,   SAMPLE     C123456              TIME  C84C
                      ORDERS

C1    URINE ROUTINE
C2    URINE CULTURE
            COLONY COUNT
            SENSITIVITY
                                           J BROWN MD
```

Fig. 16. Example of printer output resulting from a physician requesting 1) a routine urinalysis, and 2) urine culture and (antibiotic) sensitivities. This paper becomes part of the hospital medical record.

test report data entered via the 1092/1093 keyboards[*] are

transmitted directly to the central computer facility, proces-

sed, stored in the PCMR, and routed to the hospital processor

for queueing and periodic printing at appropriate nursing-

station terminals.

F. ECG; Pathology and X-Ray Systems

In each of these departments, the traditional method of

reporting the results of tests consists of the observer dictating

his findings onto magnetic tape and the contents of the tape

being transcribed to a typewritten report by a secretary. For

---

[*] Digital data is entered via the 1092/1093 keyboards as follows. (a) The appropriate keymat overlay is selected and placed up upon the keyboard — this coded form identifies to the program any given column of keys, or set of columns. The overlay keymat thus serves to identify test name and digital result variables. (b) Patient identification data, obtained from punched cards, is merged with test identification and result data and transmitted to the computer.

```
                                    DAY   113
PATIENT,   SAMPLE    C123456         TIME  1030


URINE ROUTINE       PROT = NEG     SP GR = 1.018
                    GLUC = NEG     ACET =   NEG
                                                        (a)
                    MICRO:   WBC = 0
                             RBC = RARE
                             CAST = RARE HYALINE
                             CAST = RARE GRANULAR

                                        M L BASSIS MD
```

```
                                    DAY   114
PATIENT,   SAMPLE                    TIME  1530

URINE CULTURE:    SPECIES 1 = E. COLI
                  SPECIES 2 = PROT MIRABILIS

     COLONY COUNT:    1 = >100,000/ML
                      2 = 2,500/ML

SENSITIVITY:          1 2                 1 2       (b)

           AMPICI   S R         METHIC   S R
           BACITR   R S         NALIDI   R R
           CEPHAL   R S         NEOMYC   S S
           CHLORA   R R         NITROF   S S
           GOLIST   R R         PEN G    R R
           ERYTHR   R R         STREPT   S R
           GENTAM   R S         SULFMZ   R R
           KANAM    S S         TETRA    R R

                                    M L BASSIS MD
```

Fig. 17. Examples of routine urinalysis report (a) and report of urine culture and sensitivities (b). These documents are printed by the nursing station printer and become part of the hospital medical record.

the initial phase of operation, therefore, in each of these

departments the secretaries have been supplied with an IBM

magnetic tape selectric typewriter (MT/ST) to be evaluated.
With slight modifications in her typing routine, a given secretary stores on magnetic tape the patient and test identification
data and the physician's report. These data are transmitted,
by means of a remote-record feature, to a receiver MT/ST
located in the central computer facility. By means of a Digi-
Data recorder and converter device a second tape is created
in a form acceptable for input to the center computer and
PCMR. These reports are queued and periodically transmitted to the hospital processor for routing and printing at
appropriate nursing-station terminals. This method may
eventually be replaced by terminal entry of structured data
items.

REFERENCES

1. M. F. Collen, "Periodic Health Examinations Using an
   Automated Multitest Laboratory," JAMA, 195, 830 (1966).

2. M. F. Collen, "Computer Analyses in Preventive Health
   Services," Method Inform. Med., 6, 8 (1967).

3. M. F. Collen, L. Rubin, J. Neyman, G. B. Dantzig,
   R. M. Baer, and A. B. Siegelaub, "Automated Multiphasic Screening and Diagnosis," Amer. J. Pub. Health,
   54, 741 (1964).

4. M. F. Collen, L. Rubin, and L. Davis, "Computers in
   Multiphasic Screening," Vol. 1, Chap. 14, by R. W.
   Stacy and B. D. Waxman, in Computers in Biomedical
   Research, Academic Press, New York, 1965.

5. M. F. Collen and L. F. Davis, "The Multitest Laboratory
   in Health Care," Occupational Medicine, 11, No. 7 (1969).

6. E. E. Van Brunt et al., "A Pilot Data System for a
   Medical Center," Proc. IEEE, 57, No. 11 (1969).

7. M. F. Collen, "The Multitest Laboratory in Health Care of the Future," Hospitals, 41, 119 (1967).

8. L. S. Davis, M. F. Collen, L. Rubin, and E. E. Van Brunt, "Computer Stored Medical Record," Comp. Biomed. Res., 1, 452 (1968).

7

Automation and Computerization of Clinical Laboratories

Morton D. Schwartz
Associate Professor of Electrical Engineering
California State College, Long Beach, California

I. LABORATORY AUTOMATION

The number of clinical laboratory tests is growing at the rate of 15-20% per year and has reached an estimated 1-2 billion tests during 1971 in the U.S. An estimated 575 million tests are performed in hospitals, and an additional 500 million or so in commercial laboratories. The diversity and complexity of tests are also increasing, and approximately 5-8% of the tests offered each year are new.

A. Laboratory Test Market

Assuming an average cost of $2 per test, the market for laboratory tests is $2-4 billion per year and is increasing at the rate of 15-20% per year. In order to take advantage of this potential market, several companies are currently initiating product line developments. For example, 10 companies are producing or are developing automated serum specimen analyzers. Furthermore, several additional companies are currently investigating the market potential to penetrate the field in the next 3 years.

B.   Beckman Instruments

As an example of the commitment made by some companies to penetrate the market, Beckman Instruments has spent an estimated $2 million dollars to develop its DSA-560, two-channel specimen analyzer. It was estimated by Beckman personnel that 15-30 man-years were involved over a 5-year period to complete the instrument. It is currently being offered at approximately $20,000 per system with data acquisition and teletype printout of test results. It is estimated that 100 systems must be sold before the development costs can be recovered.

The above example illustrates that a heavy commitment of resources will be required to develop automated instruments for the laboratory and that there already is considerable competition for this market.

II.   NEW INSTRUMENTS AND TESTS

In the past, the most successful types of instruments were those which were designed by laboratory workers with the cooperation and collaboration of mechanical and electrical engineers. Due to the complexity of modern semiautomated laboratory systems, industry will probably play a larger role than in the past in the design of new instruments, especially where data processing is involved in the integration of many instrument elements into a laboratory system.

Laboratory automation in the future will probably incorporate new and refined types of separation techniques including molecular separation and identification by ion exchange, gel filtration, gas chromatography, high-resolution electrophoresis, and immunoelectrophoresis [1]. Beckman Instruments is currently offering their Microzone for electrophoresis separations of serum proteins, glycoproteins, lactic dehydrogenase for isoenzyme separation, haptoglobins, hemoglobins, and immunoelectrophoresis.

A. Future Developments

Future developments will include a variety of physical, chemical, and biochemical techniques. In addition, measurements not only of blood serum, but of samples of both red cells and individual varieties of white cells will be made; and urine analysis and chemical analysis of tissues will be obtained in greater detail than any available currently.

B. Current Developments

Among the most promising current developments are the studies aimed at developing new techniques for automation and mechanization of analytic methods in frequent use. Much work remains to be done on developing techniques for deproteinization and separation of protein-free solution; for solvent extraction and separation of phases; for evaporation of solvent and concentration; for automatic centrifugation with retention of sample identity; and for discrete sample-processing methods.

C. New Test Loads

At a meeting of the Committee of Consultors [2], the group was asked to list five tests which would show the

greatest test rate growth during 1968-1973. The following were
suggested: (1) electrolytes including blood gases PO_2, PCO_2,
but not pH; (2) the SMA 12 panel; (3) enzyme and isoenzyme
pattern determinations; (4) platelet counting and liver function
tests; and (5) mono spot test and immunoelectrophoresis. It
was suggested that semiautomated equipment would be required
wherever possible to meet these requirements. Other tests
which are increasing rapidly are pregnancy tests, brain scans
by radioisotope methods, immunoelectrophoresis for newborn
screening, FTA-ADS screening for irregular antibodies in
both material groups, donors, and recipients, partial throm-
boplastin determinations, and prothrombin times.

The following tests were listed by the committee as
increasing in number during the next two years: aminoacid
analysis by automated means; immune globulin assays. It
was estimated that radioimmunodiffusion methods will greatly
increase. Also, determinations of hormones (including FSH,
estrogens, growth hormone, thyroglobulins, insulin and
certain enzymes) will greatly increase now that they can be
reliably determined by radioimmunoassay determinations
which can be made on a well counter. Enzyme determinations
by fluorometric means are being automated. Enzyme determinations in red cells (particularly those associated with
hemolytic disease), electron microscope applications of red
cell membrane defects, and identification of specific protein
components will increase as specific reagents are being
produced in greater quantity. Quantitative techniques for
specific protein components are being worked out currently.
Other tests anticipated to rise remarkably include histocom-

patibility testing for organ transplants. To date, histocompatibility testing is not very accurate, and some individuals think not really significant. Other tests on the rise include techniques for tissue analyses (not just serum analysis), instrumentation including atomic absorption and determinations of elements in very small quantities within cells.

D. Impact of Automated Instruments

The main advantages derived from large-scale introduction of autoanalyzers have been increased productivity, improved analytical performance and quality control, and lower costs when sufficient volume of tests are present. In most laboratories studied, the Technicon SMA 12's were used no more than a few hours a day. Nevertheless, cost savings were obtained; but, the potential for around-the-clock operation was never realized due to a lack of volume of tests.

E. Staffing Considerations

Staffing difficulties due to a shortage of trained medical technologists provide a justification for seriously considering centralization of a large part of the hospital service's laboratory facilities. Further system effectiveness can be obtained through the use of a core staging area within the centralized laboratory.

F. Laboratory Function Design

Functional design should incorporate control of work flow from source data and specimen collection, through emergency or routine laboratory areas, to final reporting by

the most expeditious possible routes. In general, source
material or samples should be documented and preprocessed
in a core or central assessioning area where labeling and
separating samples can be performed. Then the preprocessed
source material can be dispatched outward from the core to
the appropriate working areas by a material transport system.
Figure 1 shows a sketch of a design for such a functional
concept. An outer core is shown surrounding the core area
whose function is to provide stat capability.

III. AUTOMATION IN BIOCHEMISTRY

A. Automated Systems

If a completely automated system is defined as one
which starts with a blood sample drawn from the patient and
ends with the automatic printout of the test results along with
quality control measures and positive patient identification,
then such a system is not currently available. However,
Scientific Industries, Inc. , as described by an Arthur D.
Little report [3], is currently offering a radically new design
for a specimen analyzer that could, with the proper extensions,
fit the above definition. This new design is based on the inven-
tions of Dr. Samuel Natelson, a noted pediatric clinical
chemist. The serum sample is transferred from a micro-
capillary tube to a rectangle of filter paper mounted on a
Mylar tape and then migrates through a dialysis membrane to
another filter paper tape containing the required colorimetric
reagents. This tape is developed between heated platens and
is finally read out on a densitometer which measures reflected
light instead of the transmitted light measured with conventional wet chemistry procedures.

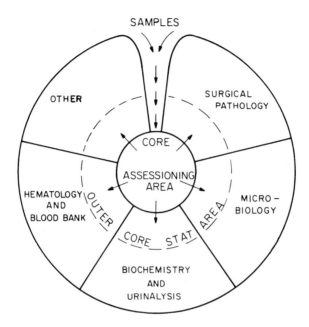

Fig. 1. Functional concept for the clinical laboratory.

Only further testing can ascertain whether the necessary accuracy and precision can be achieved with this sort of
paper-tape chemistry. If these results prove to be acceptable
then the instrument shows much potential because of its flexibility in changing over from one test to another, as well as a
very high output test rate of 360 samples per hour. Furthermore, the small sample size of one drop of serum and the
simplicity of the chemical transfer are outstanding achieve-
ments. If the instrument can be extended to include an automatic centrifuge as in the Hycel unit and a "peak picker" and
printout subsystem as in the Technicon SMA-12/30, then it
would indeed be very close to a completely automated system.

B.   Partial Systems

There are a number of partially automated analytic systems as shown in Tables I and II. The basic concept for semiautomation is one that begins with an unpipetted serum sample of approximately 3-4 ml and progresses to the final result on a strip-chart recorder. This description satisfies the versatile continuous flow system developed by Dr. Leonard Skeggs. His techniques have been widely used for a great variety of clinical chemistry determinations and have potential applications in other laboratory departments such as hematology, blood bank, and serology. For example, the Technicon SMA-7 can perform seven tests in hematology, and the Technicon Blood Typing Unit can perform blood typing and VD determinations in the blood bank.

In addition to the continuous flow system, other attempts have been made and are continuing to be made to develop partially automated systems using discrete sample processing, since the continuous flow system is protected by Technicon patents. All the instruments except for the Technicon units in Table I are discrete sample systems. The discrete handling system is closer to the manual operation and has theoretical advantages for a number of processes. Unfortunately, it also has considerable mechanical complexity.

IV.   AUTOMATION IN HEMATOLOGY

The Coulter Counter, Fisher Autocytometer and Hemalyzer, and Technicon SMA 4 and 7 are discussed in Table III and are capable of rapidly and accurately counting particles such as red cells, white cells, and platelets. These

instruments permit significant simplification of procedures in
hematology and have reduced the working time from 15 man-
minutes or more per test by the former manual methods,
which frequently produced inaccurate results, to one-fifth of
that time with consistency and reasonably good accuracy.
Nevertheless, these techniques are still semiautomatic and are
not capable of automating the sample preparation. Furthermore, the accuracy at the high and low ends of the scale can
still be improved, and the data output can be automated for
machine recording or for a data processing system.

1. Coulter Counter Model S

The Coulter Counter Model S is not shown in Table III;
however, it has been available for the past few years and is
selling for approximately $45,000. Nearly 1200 Model S's
have been sold. Its operation is similar to the Model A except
that it performs seven tests on one sample: WBC, RBC, HGB,
HCT, MCV, MCH, and MCHC. All the data are automatically
printed on test report forms or on paper tape as required.

2. Differential White Cell Count

The differential white cell counts have thus far resisted
attempts at automation. The problems of pattern recognition
have not been successfully treated by mechanical, optical,
and/or computer techniques. Current software development
will allow a single white blood cell to be classified in 7 seconds
by the computer but only after it is centered by hand in the
optical scanning field. A new approach is clearly required,
and new techniques of physical, chemical, or even enzymatic
measurement may be required.

TABLE I

Automated Instruments

Manufacturer*	Model	Approximate capital	Cost ($) per test+	Maximum hourly output samples	Number of channels#	Key Features
Technicon Corp. Ardsley, N.Y.	AutoAnalyzers SMA-12/60	61,000	0.20	60	12	Continuous flow, all liquids segmented with air bubbles, dialyzer
	SMA-7	18,000	–	60	7	Hematology – 7 tests
	Blood Typing	6,000	–	100	1	Blood typing – also VD, mononucleosis, other applications
	SMA-6/60	27,500	0.17	60	6	Basic 6-channel hospital lab analyzer
American Optical Co. (AO Instrument Co.) Richmond, Calif. (Subsidiary of Warner-Lambert)	Robot Chemist	18,400 to 21,700	0.11	120	1	Automates standard wet chemistry manipulations
AGA Corp. Oakland, Calif. (Subsidiary of AGA, Sweden)	AutoChemist	450,000	0.07	125	6-26	The most flexible, expensive, and fully automated system on the market
Beckman Instruments, Inc.	DSA-560	19,400	0.14	120	1-2	Automatic vacuum filtration of protein precipitate, all ultra-micro samples
Sherwood Medical Industries, Inc. St. Louis, Mo. (Subsidiary of Brunswick Corp.'s Health and Science Div.)	1011 Digecon	10,500 to 14,300	0.23	40	1	Semiautomatic – for intermittent use in small hospital or commercial labs

Joyce, Loebl & Co. (Subsidiary of Technical Operations) Burlington, Mass.	Mecolab	14,000	0.11	120	1-4	Manual transfers of sample racks required
DuPont (Instrument Products Div.) Wilmington, Del.	ACA	60,000-70,000	0.60-1.10	100	1-30 now; 60 possible	Ion exchange or gel filtration for protein separation – novel plastic bag forms precision optical cell
Hycel, Inc. Houston, Texas	Mark X	1,250/mo	0.14	40	10	Push-button programming, automatic centrifuge; select any or all of 10 tests per sample
Scientific Industries, Inc. Hempstead, N.Y.	MSAS/360	9,000	0.10	360	1	Microsamples – densitometer read-out of color reactions on paper tape
Bausch & Lomb, Inc. Rochester, N.Y.	Zymat 340	10,000	0.40	25	1	For enzymes only, very precise

* Listed in approximate order of market entry.

+ Average materials and labor only, assuming technologist salary of $6000 per year, one-shift operation, and 50% efficiency (due to the need for standards, controls, blanks, etc.). Cost per test does not include set-up time, which is very important for short runs.

Tests per sample.

M. D. SCHWARTZ

TABLE II

Automatic Chemistry Machines at Denver AACC Show (August 1969)

Company	Machine	ch#/sam-ples/hr.	Total samp/size	I.D.	Output	Comments on I.D. scheme
Beckman	DSA-560	2/120	Micro	Sequence from work list	?	?
AGA	Autochemist	24/135	6 ml	Rack No. reader	PDP-8, TTY ASR33	Rack No. is recorded on patient ID card when sample is placed in rack
Vickers	Multichannel 300	20/300	6 ml	Vial No. reader	PDP-8, TTY ASR33	Container vial is designed for machine/eyeball reading. System requires hand encoding
Hycell	Mark X	10/40	Macro	Sequence from work list	Chart like Technicon	Programmed reagent dispensing – operator must tie chart No. to sample No. to patient sample. Stat cups break sequence.
Perkin-Elmer	C-4	4/30	350 λ	Vial No. reader	Printed tape	Requisition (IBM stub) tag on sample cup. Transfer from vacutainer, centrifuge
Union Carbide	Centrifichem	1/120	50 λ	Sequence from work list	Printed tape	All cuvettes continuously sampled by spinning disk past photometer
DuPont	ACA	1-30/100	Macro	Vial No. printed	Printed tape	ID label is photographed onto result sheet. ID attached to sample cup at machine
Clay Adams	—	?/?	Macro	Vacutainer reader	DVM (or tape?)	If centrifuge is built in, then no ID mixup possible in lab
Technicon	SMA	12/60	Macro	Sequence from work list	Chart	Chart No. to sample No. to patient sample
Smith Kline	Eska Lab	?	?	?	?	?

3. Coagulation Procedures

Other areas in hematology that use tests essentially chemical in nature such as coagulation procedures, have been partially automated. Several instruments are currently available, such as the Ames Sera Tek Prothrombin Time System, Bio-Quest Fibrometer System Coagulation Timer, Adams Thrombitron, Coleman Prothrombin Timer, Haemoscope Thrombelastograph, Modern Laboratory Chronothrombin Oxford Prothromter, Phipps Prothrombin Test Bath, and Sanborn Coagulation Analyzer. All of the instruments are semiautomated and employ detectors to measure a change in conductivity caused by the formation of fibrin gel across electrodes or a change in optical density, as light is transmitted through a blood or plasma sample.

V. LABORATORY DATA PROCESSING

A. Processing Time

At present, apart from the time spent on the chemical analysis itself, most of the time required by a laboratory to process a request for chemical investigation derives from the following: (1) from the initial clerical work relating to the request form itself, and (2) from the various steps which are primarily of a clerical nature between the completion of the chemical processes of analysis and issue of the final result from the laboratory in the form of a report.

Attempts at reducing the work involved in dealing with the requests have been studied [4]. To further simplify the work load, some companies have incorporated into their

TABLE III

Automatic Cell Counter*

Manufacturer and address	Blood Cell counter	Principle	Type of receptor and circuit	Counting range (standard dilution) RBC million/cmm	WBC thousand cmm	Measurable particle sizes microns
Coulter Electronics, Inc. 590 West 20th Street Hialeah, Florida 33010	Coulter Counter Model A	Based on electrical conductivity differences between all blood cells and common diluents; blood cells are insulators, diluents good conductors	Solid state amplifier, digital voltmeter	0-7.5	0-50	1-20
	Coulter Counter Model D-2	Same as for Model A above	Solid state amplifier, digital voltmeter	0-7.5	0-50	1-20
	Coulter Counter Model F	Same as for Model A above	Solid state amplifier, digital voltmeter	0-7.5	0-50	1-20
Fisher Scientific Co. 711 Forbes Ave. Pittsburgh, Pa. 15219	Autocytometer	Light-scattering photometer	Photomultiplier, meter	0-7.5	0-15	1-50
	Hemalyzer	Light-scattering photometer	Photomultiplier digital printout	0-9.99	0-99.99	1-50
Technicon Corp. Ardsley, N.Y. 10502	SMA-4 SMA-7	Dark field optical, light-scattering	Photomultiplier, solid state signal circuits, read-out in cell concentrations	0-8.0	0-25	2-30

Company	Model							Comments
Coulter Electronics, Inc. 590 West 20th Street Hialeah, Florida 33010	A	1:50,000	1:500	±1.0	±3.2	?	15	Oscilloscope for complete system checkout
	D-2	1:50,000	1:500	±1.0	±3.2	?	15	Does not permit cell size distribution studies
	F	1:50,000	1:500	±1.0	±3.2	?	15	Oscilloscope for complete system checkout; orifice image display for optical aperture checkout
Fisher Scientific Co. 711 Forbes Ave. Pittsburgh, Pa. 15219	Autocytometer	1:62,500	1:250	±0.75	±1.5	0.75	35	
	Hemalyzer	1:62,500	1:250	±2.5 S.D.	±4.2 S.D.	20 lambda whole blood	96 secs	Does Hemoglobin and provides digital presentation of results on tape
Technicon Corp. Ardsley, N.Y. 10502	SMA/4 SMA/7	1:10,000	1:40	2.0 C.V.	3.1 C.V.	?	60 samples/hr	Automatic sampling and dilution; built-in oscilloscope; measures RBC, WBC, Hgb, Hct, plus three erythrocyte constants (SMA-7)

* Summarized in part from Laboratory Management series on new instruments 1969.

instruments the capability for data processing. For example, the SMA 12 draws out the test results as an analog trace across a calibrated chart. The data can be further processed by an Infotronics unit to provide punched paper tape for computer record keeping or telephone transmission to remote facilities.

B. Laboratory Computers

In order to reduce the estimated one-third of the medical technologist's time spent in record keeping or clerical tasks, several companies have introduced computer systems for data acquisition and processing. Table IV shows 51 laboratories with computerized equipment. These computer systems are primarily designed to collect data in an on-line mode from the autoanalyzer channels and compute the test results. Several designs, such as those of BSL and DNA, allow for manual inputs of data from the laboratory work areas by desk-top terminals tied to a laboratory computer. Table V provides several examples of some of the earliest laboratories which have used laboratory computers.

VI. AUTOMATION IN MICROBIOLOGY

The least progress in automation has been made in microbiology, except for the area of serologic reactions where continuous flow techniques offer considerable promise. Techniques in microbiology, such as isolation of bacteria, counting of bacteria in urine and other fluids, and antibiotic sensitivity testing, are potentially susceptible to automation. Some efforts along these lines are already in progress. A NIH concept for automated sensitivity testing with rapid turn around has been developed to the prototype stage, but is not being pursued any further due to a lack of clinical interest in the device.

The whole field of microbiology offers one of the most fruitful opportunities for improved efficiency, accuracy, and rapidity of obtaining useful laboratory data for direct patient care and research. There are several basic biochemical and physiochemical methods which could be developed and applied toward automating the fields of bacteriology, serology, and virology.

VII. AUTOMATION IN BLOOD BANK

The automation of blood bank functions must be made absolutely error proof before it can replace present manual techniques for cross matching. Continuous flow techniques are being developed, and Technicon is offering for $6000 a semiautomated system for blood typing and VDRL applications.

The cross matching of blood for transfusions is extremely difficult to automate because of the nature of the problem itself and the very high order of accuracy and reliability required. However, some of the quantitative procedures in blood banking such as agglutination reactions are susceptible to improved instrumental techniques.

VIII. COST-EFFECTIVENESS STUDIES

Several studies have been performed to provide economic justification for clinical laboratory automation and computerization. One of the most extensive studies started in 1968 by a study group formed in Minneapolis and comprised of

TABLE IV

Computerized Clinical Laboratories

Item	Institution	Status		Off-line	On-line			
		In Dev.	In Oper.	Noncomputer data acquisition system	Small computer systems	Medium computer systems	Med.-large computer systems	Small computers linked to large computers
1.	University of Tennessee	X		IBM 1080				
2.	Firestone Hospital (Akron, O.)	X		IBM 1080				
3.	Notre Dame Hospital (Montreal)	X		IBM 1080				
4.	Youngstown	X		IBM 1080	IBM 1130			
5.	Clinical Lab Group (Los Angeles)	X			IBM 1130 & PDP 12	IBM 360/30		
6.	Methodist Hospital (Brooklyn)	X			PDP8/S			
7.	New England Priv. Res. Cntr.	X			PDP8/S			
8.	Wake Forest	X			PDP8/S			
9.	University of Virginia				PDP8			
10.	Mason Clinic (Seattle)	X			PDP8			
11.	Lab Procedures/Upjohn Corp. (Culver City, Calif.)	X			PDP8 (Outputs to 360 compatible magnetic tape, tape off-line to 360/30)			
12.	Kaiser Permanente (S.F. - Oakland)	X					Autochemi (Includes PDP8)-link to IBM 360/50 planned	
13.	Biosciences Laboratories (Van Nuys, Calif.)	X			2-LINC 8's and 2-PDP 15's			
14.	Duke University (Durham, N.C.)	X			2-LINC8's			
15.	University of Wisconsin	X			LINC8			
16.	University of California Medical Center (San Francisco)	X			BSL			
17.	Perth Amboy	X			Spear-LINC			
18.	University of Colorado	X				IBM 1800		
19.	University of Kentucky	X				IBM 1800		
20.	University of Washington		X			IBM 1800		
21.	King County Med Labs (Seattle)	X				IBM 1800		
22.	Presbyterian-St. Luke's (Chicago)	X			BSL			
23.	St. Vincent Hospital (Portland)	X			BSL			
24.	Medical College South Carolina	X			BSL			
25.	Harrisburg Hosp. (Harrisburg, Penn.)	X			BSL			
26.	Meyer Memorial Hosp. (Buffalo, N.Y.)	X			BSL			
27.	Meriden Hosp. (Meriden, Conn.)	X			BSL			

No.	Institution	A	B	Computer(s)
28.	Metropolitan Lab (Teneack, N.J.)		X	BSL
29.	University of British Columbia	X		PDP 9
30.	Latter Day Saints Hospital (Salt Lake City)		X	CDC 3200, 3300; PDP8; 360/65
31.	University of Minnesota	X		CDC 3200
32.	North Memorial Hosp. (Minneapolis)		X	DNA
33.	University of Kansas		X	BSL
34.	University of Alberta		X	BSL
35.	University of Missouri		X	IBM 1440
36.	Veterans Administration Hospital (L.A.)		X	Honeywell 516 and 1200
37.	Army Nutritional Center (Fitzsimmons Army Hosp., Colo.)	X		Infotronics
38.	City of Memphis Hospital		X	IBM 1080
39.	Yale New Haven		X	IBM 1130
40.	Sutter Commun. & Gen. Hosp. (Sacramento, Calif.)		X	Spear-LINC; IBM 360/40
41.	Methodist Hospital of Brooklyn		X	PDP8
42.	Hennepin County Gen. Hospital (Minneapolis)		X	DNA
43.	Mercy Hospital (Urbana, Illinois)		X	LINC 8
44.	Ohio State Hospital (Columbus, Ohio)		X	LINC 8
45.	Teishin Hospital (Tokyo, Japan)		X	LINC 8
46.	Framingham Union Hospital (Framingham, Massachusetts)		X	LINC 8
47.	Conemaugh Valley Memorial Hospital (Johnstown, Pennsylvania)		X	PDP 12
48.	United Medical Lab (Portland, Oregon)		X	BSL, IBM 1800, IBM 360
49.	Massachusetts General Hospital		X	PDP8/S (2) Coulter Counter Systems; PDP-9 (2)
50.	Saskatchewan, U., Canada		X	Spear-LINC
51.	Luthern General & Deaconess Hosps. (Park Ridge, Ill.)	X		DNA

members from the systems and programs group of Minnesota
Hospital Services Association and pathologists and chief technologists from 10 participating hospitals in the Minneapolis-
St. Paul area.   The purpose of this study was to determine the
economic feasibility of laboratory data processing systems.

A.   First Phase

The first phase of the study was to determine the feasibility of a large central computer system to be shared by these
participating hospital laboratories.   With such a system, test
results from each laboratory would be sent over telephone
lines to the central computer where test results can be com-
piled.   Completed reports would be generated by a printer
located in each laboratory.

The results of the study indicated that lack of standardization in clinical laboratories, the need for immediate verification of test results, plus the cost to develop such a centralized system, made this approach economically unfeasible.

B.   Second Phase

The second phase was to perform an economic feasibility study based on the use of a dedicated laboratory computer
in each laboratory.   This phase required an accurate labor
cost per test analysis based on several prior years of previous
operation.   Projections were made for the next 5 years with
respect to the increased number of tests anticipated plus the
increase in personnel who would be needed to handle this
projected test volume.

TABLE V

Examples of Early Computerized Laboratories*

Place	Subject	Type of Automation	Computer
San Francisco General Hospital Dr. M. Pollycove Dr. M. Fish	Laboratory organization. Projected use of PDP8 and BSL equipment in chemical laboratories.	Laboratory on-line operation.	PDP8 and BSL equipment.
University of Colorado Medical School, Denver Dr. E. B. Reeve Dr. Aikawa	Use of computers in physiological measurements. Data processing in routine hospital laboratories.	Multiple and single-channel AutoAnalyzers on-line to IBM 1800.	On-line data processing using IBM 1800.
Department of Clinical Pathology, Northside Hospital, Youngstown Hospitals Association, Ohio Dr. A. E. Rappoport Mr. W. Gennaro	Use of IBM 1080 system.	IBM 1080 Patient Identification system in use in certain areas of the laboratory.	IBM 1080 combined with a manual punching system. Results fed off-line to an IBM 360/30. IBM 1050 duplicating cards fed in from Youngstown Southside Hospital.
Sutter Community & General Hospitals, Sacramento, Calif.	Laboratory data management.	AutoAnalyzers on-line.	Spear-LINC Class 300
Army Nutritional Center, Colorado		AutoAnalyzers on-line. Gas chromatograph on-line.	Infotronics and PDP8/S.
Clinical Pathology Dept. National Institutes of Health, Bethesda, Md. Dr. G. Z. Williams Dr. E. Cotlove Dr. D. Young Dr. T. Dutcher Dr. Marsh	Use of on-line computer facilities in laboratories. Laboratory organization. Accuracy and precision. Use of large laboratory computer. Specimen identification. Biochemical individuality. Development of an automatic enzyme analyzer. Automation of bacteriology.	A six channel system of AutoAnalyzers on-line to a CDC 3200 computer. A patient-specimen identification system (not fully mechanized). A discrete enzyme analyzer based on the Gilford Record Spectrophotometer. Experimental apparatus to log bacterial growth by turbidity for antibiotic testing.	Use of punched card requesting with computer output of worksheets and reports. Limited statistical evaluations of laboratory findings. Berkeley Scientific Laboratories data console used for input of hematological results to the computer. Paper or magnetic tape as buffer store.

Place	Subject	Type of Automation	Computer
Los Angeles County-USC Medical Center Dr. A. G. Ware	Laboratory organization. Division of the laboratory into (a) routine (b) emergency and (c) special investigation areas.	Prototype of a Beckman 4-channel discrete automatic analyzer.	Ties into central IBM 360 County Hospital system.
Bio-Science Laboratories, Van Nuys, Calif. Dr. R. H. Henry Dr. G. Kessler	Organization of a large commercial laboratory.	AutoAnalyzers on-line to IBM 1800 for initial system. Currently using LINC 8's and PDP 15's.	Cards punched with results (a) from manual tests by key-punching and (b) from AutoAnalyzers by IBM 1800 on-line. All cards then fed to IBM 1440 computer for billing and records.
School of Medicine, University of California-Los Angeles Mr. W. S. Russell Prof. P. Sturgeon	Use of data processing in clinical chemistry and surgical histology. Use of continuous flow techniques in hematology.	Use of the AutoAnalyzer in serology.	IBM 360/75 installation to record surgical pathology findings. Routine storage and reporting of biochemical results.
Perth Amboy General Hospital, New Jersey Dr. H. C. Pribor and Dr. W. R. Kirkham Pathologists Mr. J. Foley and Dr. G. Fellows of the Spear Corporation	The use of the Spear Computer System in a laboratory serving a 550 bed general hospital, including the potential of the system for further development.	Technicon equipment: SMA-12 Survey Model and various AutoAnalyzer units in routine use; SMA-4 in use in hematology.	The Spear system. Some routine use of the computer, e.g., for protein electrophoresis calculations.
Section of Clinical Pathology, School of Medicine, Yale University, New Haven, Conn.	Laboratory automation and data processing.	A series of laboratory-built discrete analyzers all linked to one data logger.	Cards from the data logger processed in an IBM 1130 sited in the laboratory and operated by laboratory technicians.

King's County Research Laboratories, Brooklyn, New York Mr. M. A. Blaivas Mr. A. Mencz	Organization of a large commercial laboratory receiving specimens by van delivery from practitioners and small hospitals from the New York area and by post from much of the USA and from other countries.	Multiple AutoAnalyzers on-line to a computer.	AutoAnalyzers on-line to an IBM 1710 computer. Replacement of this by an IBM 1800 data acquisition system was well advanced and an IBM 360/30 computer is then to be used for data processing and billing.
Division of Clinical Pathology and Laboratory Medicine, University of California, San Francisco Dr. G. Brecher Dr. O. Siggaard-Anderson	Use of PDP8 computer and Berkeley Scientific Laboratories (BSL) equipment in hematology and chemical laboratories. Microanalysis.	Several microtechniques devised by Dr. Siggaard-Anderson.	Routine use of PDP8 and BSL laboratory data input consoles, mainly for hematology.
Montreal, Prov. of Quebec, Canada Dr. M. Young (Toronto) Mr. E. Whitehead, Technicon Instruments Corp. Dr. G. Letellier, Hospital Notre-Dame, Montreal	Inpatient and outpatient screening techniques. Accuracy and precision of the SMA-12. Specimen identification and off-line data processing.	SMA-12 coupled to IBM 1080 system.	Cards from IBM 1080 transmitted by IBM 1050 to IBM 1130 computer several miles away.
Permanente Medical Group Medical Methods Research Oakland, California Dr. S. Ramcharan	Clinical and laboratory testing of ambulant population.	Specially built 8-channel AutoAnalyzer and various devices for rapid clinical measurements. Currently using AutoChemists from AGA Corporation.	Signals from AutoAnalyzer converted to a result and punched automatically into cards. Anthropometric measurements also automatically punched into cards. Other data entered on cards by mark-sensing. All cards processed by IBM 360/40. IBM 2701 system receiving signals from cards read at a remote station and transmitting directly into the computer.

* Summarized in part from survey performed by Dr. T. P. Whitehead, United Kingdom Ministry of Health Survey of North American Laboratories.

Estimates of the clerical time saved that would be achieved through the use of a dedicated laboratory computer system were determined. The clerical time saved would reduce the number of additional personnel needed for the projected increased volume. These cost savings for future personnel were compared to the cost of a $150,000 laboratory computer system prorated over a 5-year period.

This phase of the study was performed by each hospital using the hospital controller and the laboratory pathologist. While the results varied from hospital to hospital, they can be interpreted to indicate that a hospital with 400 beds or more could economically justify the use of a dedicated laboratory computer. These results imply that effective laboratory management would be required to modify the operation of the laboratory to take advantage of clerical time saved. The hospitals studied varied in bed size with the smallest hospital studied being 161 beds.

C.   Third Phase

The third phase of the study will be an evaluation of the existing laboratory computer systems on the market in an effort to select one system which would best meet the needs of this group of hospitals.

IX.   DEDICATED LABORATORY COMPUTER SYSTEMS

Several dedicated laboratory computer systems are currently available. Some of these systems are: Berkeley Scientific Laboratories Systems (BSL); IBM 1800 and 1080

Data Acquisition and Control Systems; Spear Clinical Laboratory System; Infotronics; CLINILAB from Digital Equipment Corp. (DEC); and, Diversified Numeric Applications (DNA). Applications of these systems are summarized in the next chapter, where a more detailed description of each system is provided.

REFERENCES

1. T. D. Kinney, and R. S. Melville, "Automation in Clinical Laboratories," Laboratory Investigation, 16, No. 5, 803 (1967).

2. Notes made from Committee of Consultors Meeting, February 1968.

3. Arthur D. Little, "Automation in the Clinical Laboratory – Five New Competitors," October 7, 1968.

4. S. Lee, and I. Schoen, "Quality Control Aspects of the Chemistry Laboratory Form," Amer. J. Clinical Path., 47, No. 3, 329 (1967).

8

Computing Systems in Hospital Laboratories

Marion J. Ball
Assistant Professor, Department of Medical Physics
John C. Ball
Professor, Department of Psychiatry
and
Eugene A. Magnier
Director of Computing Center
Temple University
Philadelphia, Pennsylvania

I. INTRODUCTION

This chapter is a summary of the state of the art of computer applications in the clinical laboratory in the United States in 1969. It is a good example of the ever-active and rapid rate of development in the medical computing field. The area of clinical laboratory computerization has had several new vendor entries during the past few years, and the long-term vendors have modified and changed many basic procedures. More up-to-date and expanded presentations on this topic can be found in: Selecting a Computer System for the Clinical Laboratory, by M. J. Ball, Charles C. Thomas, Springfield, 1971, and Clinical Laboratory Computer Systems, A Comprehensive Evaluation, prepared for the College of American Pathologists, by J. Lloyd Johnson Associates, Northbrook, Illinois, 1971.

The rapidly increasing workload in the clinical laboratories in most American hospitals has resulted in an acute shortage of trained technologists. One way to alleviate this shortage is to relieve them of their clerical duties and let them work more in the areas for which they are trained. Manual errors in calculating results are another problem in most laboratories. Although straight-line interpolation and visual estimating of strip charts are often inaccurate, it is impractical for the ordinary technologist to use a more sophisticated statistical method of determining results manually (e. g. , second-degree curve fitting and interpolation). There are also problems involved in transfer of data from one document to another.

This leads one to ask how many of these problems can be solved by computerization of the pathology clinical laboratory? Although laboratory requirements are often quite diverse and the output from the several operational computer systems are not uniform, the following advantages have been realized in many automated clinical laboratories: (1) more rapid reporting of test results, (2) reduction of clerical error, (3) improved legibility, and (4) a unified and updated report of the laboratory tests performed for each patient.

The extent of improvement to be realized by computerization is related to the size and complexity of the pathology laboratory; it is most directly associated with the amount of work performed. Thus, computerization is most likely to be rewarding in large pathology laboratories with a considerable volume of work. In this regard, it is important to keep in mind that the principal advantages derived from installation of a computer system occur after the pathology tests have been performed; it provides a rapid and accurate means of combining, reporting, filing, and retrieving test results. While a computer system may reduce the time required to perform a specific test, particularly if manual calculations are required, the main advantage of computerization is the improvement effected by the systematic organization of the laboratory test results into an accessible data bank.

The aim of this chapter is to evaluate nine approaches to the automation of a pathology laboratory. Each of the systems to be reviewed are presently in operation, and all have been seen by at least one of the authors (see Tables I and II). The nine systems described are the following.

(1) A general batch processing procedure, computer not in the laboratory.

(2) A general batch processing procedure, computer in the laboratory.

(3) The International Business Machines 1800 Data Acquisition and Control System (IBM 1800).

(4) The International Business Machines 1080 Data Acquisition System with Automated Chemistry Programs (IBM 1080). The IBM 1080 System was actually withdrawn from the market by IBM in the fall of 1970. The approach, however, is being considered by other vendors such as Info-Med, in Princeton, New Jersey.

TABLE I

Basic Characteristics of Nine Computer Systems

	BSL	DEC	DNA	Infotronics	IBM batch processing	IBM 1130	IBM 1800	IBM 1080	Spear
On-line capabilities	Yes	Yes	Yes	Yes	No	Yes	Yes	Yes	Yes
Off-line capabilities	Yes	Yes	Yes	Yes	Yes	Yes	Yes	Yes	Yes
Immediate access capability	Yes	Yes	Yes	Yes	No	Yes	Yes	No	Yes
Special console terminals	Yes	No	Yes	No	No	No	No	No	Yes
Turn-key system	Yes	Yes	Yes	Yes	No	No	No	No	Yes
Computer in the laboratory	Yes	Yes	Yes	Yes	No	Yes	Yes	No	Yes
More than five installations	Yes	Yes	No	No	Yes	Yes	Yes	Yes	Yes
Free English text options	No	Yes	No	Yes	Yes	Yes	Yes	No	Yes
Coded messages	Yes	Yes	Yes	Yes	Yes	Yes	Yes	No	Yes

TABLE II

Characteristics of Nine Computer Systems

	BSL	DEC	DNA	Info-tronics	IBM batch processing	IBM 1130	IBM 1800	IBM 1080	Spear
I. Data output equipment									
A. Teletype	Yes	Yes	Yes	Yes	No	No	No	No	Yes
B. Kleinschmidt printer	Yes	No	No	No	No	No	No	No	Yes
C. Line printer	Yes	Yes	Yes	No	Yes	Yes	Yes	No	Yes
D. Cathode ray tube (output option)	No	No	No	No	No	No	No	No	Yes
II. Data input equipment									
A. Mark-sense cards	Yes	No	No	No	No	No	Yes	No	Yes
B. Porta-punch cards	No	No	No	No	Yes	Yes	Yes	Yes	Yes
C. Terminals									
1. Keyboard entry	Yes	No	Yes	No	No	Yes	No	No	No
2. Cathode ray tube remote entry	No	No	No	No	No	No	No	No	Yes
3. Cathode ray tube at CPU (graphic display)	Yes	Yes	No	Yes	No	No	No	No	Yes
4. Teletype									
a. Terminal	No	Yes	No	Yes	No	No	No	No	No
b. At CPU	Yes	Yes	Yes	Yes	No	No	No	No	Yes
III. Cost									
A. Rent	Yes	No	No	No	Yes	Yes	Yes	Yes	Yes
B. Lease	Yes	Yes	Yes	Yes	Yes	Yes	Yes	Yes	Yes
C. Purchase price (in thousands)*	140	150	175	120	**	**	250	**	130

*All prices quoted above are only very general approximations and should not be cited as actual price.

**See Clinical Laboratory Computer Systems, a Comprehensive Evaluation, J. Lloyd Johnson Associates, Northbrook, 1971 for current pricing information.

(5)   The Berkeley Scientific Laboratories Clin-Data
      and Chem-Data Systems (BSL).

(6)   The Digital Equipment Clinical Laboratory System
      (LABCOM 4 and Clini-Lab 12).

(7)   The B-D Spear Clinical Laboratory Automation
      System (CLAS-300).

(8)   Infotronics 3055.

(9)   Diversified Numeric Applications (division of
      Avnet, Inc.) (DNA).

Before describing and evaluating these nine computer
systems, however, it is pertinent to discuss several basic
concepts of computerization.

II.   LABORATORY COMPUTER CHARACTERISTICS

A.   Hardware and Software

The difficulties encountered in computerizing pathology
laboratories are problems of management and programming
rather than of machine deficiencies. Both the machine, the
overall commands, and the design of the system (i.e., the
software), are important. There is a tendency, however, to
overemphasize the capabilities of the machine and to under-
estimate the management function, which is only provided by
the software. It is easy to sell machines. It is less apparent
that the intelligibility and correctness of the message or
instructions is equally important.

One basic way of considering computer systems and
clarifying their capabilities is to separate the machine from
the instructions it receives — the hardware from the software.

The hardware includes the central processing and storage machines or units, as well as the input and output units. The term "hardware" refers to the machines themselves, the physical part of the computer system. The term "software" refers to the coded instructions (i. e. , programs) given to the computer to determine how the computer handles a task and in what form the computer will present the results (i. e. , output). The software, therefore, performs the management function without which the actual hardware would be of little use. Instructions are issued to the hardware in the form of written computer languages such as machine language, assembly language, FORTRAN, and PL/I. The process of coding instructions into a computer language, that is, a language that a particular computer will accept and act upon, is called programming.

B. On-Line Versus Off-Line or Batch Processing Systems

Two distinct approaches have been taken in automating the clinical pathology laboratory, those of on-line and off-line procedures.

An operation is said to be off-line (i. e. , a batch system), if data from or to the laboratory instrument is not directly controlled by the computer. When a sufficient amount of data is accumulated it is then transported to the computer for processing according to either the workload or a pre-determined schedule. At times, an off-line system may increase the initial clinical workload since in establishing the source record basic patient information, test results, etc. , must be keypunched or entered by way of a key-stroke operation. The reward, however, for the extra effort is that the computer now has the resource in its data bank to report with more accuracy and speed the laboratory test results to the clinics, wards, and physicians with the elimination of the many clerical errors generated by repeated hand data transcriptions.

An on-line real-time computer process is one in which the data is fed directly into the computer from the laboratory instrument with no human intervention in the recording of test results. Since there is no appreciable time lag between the operation of the laboratory instrument and that of the computer the process is said to be "real-time."

The distinct advantage, however, of an on-line system is that electronic interfacing modules attached to such instruments as autoanalyzers and Coulter Counters directly transfer data into the computer. Manual keypunching is, therefore, eliminated and the possibility of error greatly reduced.

With the on-line system, the machine takes over many of the tasks which were previously performed by the technologist. For example, the computer can take the results from an autoanalyzer, pick the peak, give the peak a numeric value, interpolate against standards, and record the result on the internal laboratory report form, and transfer the final result via a terminal directly to the nursing station. These four functions can be handled on-line by the computer. The end results can be retrieved in multiple and varied format, such as per patient tests, alphabetic listings, or tests by hospital number or ward location. This is a programming function.

Even installations that have on-line capabilities at the
present usually supplement the data acquisition with manual
inputs from the laboratories doing their work off-line. The
University of Kentucky Clinical Pathology Department, for
example, has most of the general chemistry area on-line,
but enters the hematology results into the computer by way of
cards (i. e. , batch) [9].

The most common on-line equipment at present are
the single, dual, SMA-7A and SMA-12/60 type autoanalyzers,
Coulter Counter, the Beckman 560, and the Coulter S. Eventually, it would be desirable if most clinical laboratory
equipment were directly connected into a central processor.

C. Immediate Access versus Closed Shop

The term "immediate access" refers to the prompt
availability of data stored in a central processing unit. To
have immediate access to computer storage requires special
effort and hardware designed with interrupt capabilities.
Immediate access in this field can be obtained only in a
"dedicated" computer environment, one in which the computer
deals exclusively with data from a single area (in this case,
the pathology laboratory). The computer must be present in
the laboratory. A pathologist may then request information
from the computer at will. Technically, immediate access
can be had in shared systems. Practically, this has not been
successful.

1. Example of Immediate Access

The request for immediate data can be entered into the system by way of a variety of inputs such as a teletype or typewriter terminal. For example, a telephone call from Ward B comes to the laboratory; the doctor would like to know whether or not Mary Smith's blood sugar, glucose, and electrolytes have been run. With a computer system which has immediate access capabilities in the laboratory, the technologist or machine operator enters a prescribed code into the computer requesting the above information. Almost instantaneously, in some 2 seconds, the answer will be printed on one of the on-line printers or appear on a cathode ray display tube (CRT). This unit could be located at the nursing station or in the laboratory.

It must be kept in mind, however, that immediate access as described above can be available only for information that has been stored in the computer memory. For example, information on laboratory tests run for the past 4 days would be immediately accessible; information on laboratory tests performed 3 years ago would not. The recent laboratory information would reside on an "on-call" access device and the time lapse between request and response would be only that time required for the machine operator to enter the request plus time required for the printer to print out the desired information (or for it to appear on the CRT). Information on tests performed 3 years ago would be stored outside of computer memory and the time lapse between request and response would include time in which the machine operator would have to mount a tape or stored disc to make the requested information available to the computer, in addition to the time required for entering the final request and printout.

2. Example of Closed Shop

In contrast, a computer system operating on a "closed shop" basis is one in which "all computer programming, coding, and operating functions are performed by members of a regular computing staff. The operation of a computing facility where programming service to the user is the responsibility of a group of specialists, thereby effectively separating the phase of task formulation from that of computer implementation. The programmers are not allowed in the computer room to run or oversee the running of their programs. " The computer here is used by a wide variety of departments; the first job may be from the physics department, the second from the admitting office, the third from the sociology department, and so on. The jobs are logged at the computing center, run, and the output then returned to the user at a later time.

Obviously there is a distinct advantage in having patient information, test results, statistics, etc., available on request. In order to effect the immediate access capability most beneficially the need for special training and organization must be emphasized [16].

D. Down-Time Considerations

One of the major concerns of the clinical laboratory director and the pathologists who use the laboratory is the

importance of getting the laboratory test results out on time:
this is one of the initial reasons for installation of a computer
system. The reliability of the system to maintain the quality
of service demanded is therefore a most important consideration for the user. The question is will the system always
operate?

The laboratory director must be aware of the varieties
of "down-time," or time in which the computer is not functioning. Preventive maintenance is planned down-time which
can be scheduled when the laboratory is not functioning at
peak periods. Unplanned down-time, or breakdowns, is of
much greater concern. Breakdowns can be caused by malfunc-
tion of the central processing unit, a software-programming
error, air-conditioning failures, input device failure, output
device failure, or simply an electrical failure. All of these
emergencies should be taken into consideration and a well-
planned backup system made available. It is worth considering
the desirability of a periodic day of hand processing, once a
month possibly, in order to maintain the ability to process
laboratory results independent of the computer.

E. Specimen Identification

One of the paramount problems encountered in all
clinical laboratory systems is that of the correct identification
of test results — the problem of identifying the patient for
whom the test was performed. Two system solutions are in
common use [2, 4, 6]. The first is the IBM 1084 Sample
Reader, part of the IBM 1080 System and designed for use

with laboratory instruments which supply the sipping device.
The second is the generation of a separate work list for each
autoanalyzer (i. e. , for each test).   This informs the technologist of the order in which the serum cups should be entered
on the autoanalyzer tray.   This procedure establishes a one-
to-one relationship between the test results and the patient.

III. COMPUTER SYSTEM REVIEW

Each review will include the following: (1) a brief
description of the system including hardware and software,
input and output devices (terminals); (2) on-line real-time or
off-line batch processing capabilities; (3) immediate access
capabilities; (4) a listing of hospitals in which each system is
installed; and (5) advantages and limitations of each system
as seen by the authors.

A.   Central Computer Remote from Laboratory

A central computer approach is the most general
application being used in pathology laboratories.   In this case
a central computer which is not in the laboratory is employed
on a batch process closed-shop basis.   In a batch processing
approach the laboratory results are punched into cards.   After
a sufficient number of cards have been amassed they are
carried to a computer facility.   Then, according to the workload at the computer center or a prearranged schedule, the
cards are sorted in proper sequence and run through the
computer.   The resultant output (the desired information) is
then returned to the laboratory.

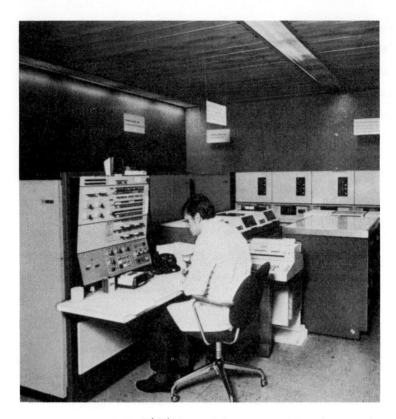

Fig. 1. The IBM 360/40 used for general batch processing procedures.

In this batch processing procedure a centrally located
computer is employed on a "closed-shop" basis. Thus, the
batch processing system addresses itself mainly to the
reporting problem of the laboratory. It has neither on-line
data collection capabilities nor immediate recall capabilities
(see Fig. 1).

Comments. A basic problem with batch processing
is that the computer facility and the clinical laboratory are

usually under different management and control. Thus the
laboratory staff is attempting to complete and distribute test
results as rapidly and accurately as possible while the computer staff may have other tasks to which they must attend as
well as a different order of priority. The end result is that
it is often difficult or impossible for the clinical laboratory
to obtain the necessary output at the time it is needed.

If suitable cooperation with a computer center can be
established, the batch processing approach can be quite
successful. Dr. Rappaport at the Youngstown (Ohio) Hospital
has succeeded for this reason. Not only does he have financial
and administrative control over the clinical laboratory, but
his unit is a major financial contributor to the hospital computing center, and, therefore, can demand a high priority on
service rendered. Dr. Rappaport used the ACP (Automated
Chemistry Program), on the 360/30, 2 hours daily at the rate
of $100 per hour; this cost does not include the 1080 Data
Acquisition System located in the laboratory [13]. (Cost
figures on large and small computers can be found in Mathews'
report [10].)

Other batch processing procedures are successfully
employed by Dr. Straumfjord [15] at the University of
Alabama Medical School, Dr. Finley [3] at Fairview Hospital, Minneapolis, Minnesota, and Dr. Goldblatt [18] at
Conemaugh Valley Memorial Hospital in Johnstown, Pennsylvania. These physicians were among the first to computerize
their pathology laboratories in the United States. It must be
realized, however, that these laboratories are limited in that

their reports are generated from punched cards and require
a large clerical and secretarial staff.

B. Laboratory Computer

One alternative to the use of separate computer facilities is to install a small computer system in one's own laboratory. This has worked successfully in a number of hospitals
with an IBM 1130, for example. The advantage of such a
dedicated computer facility is that one is not dependent on
outside cooperation. Furthermore, one can utilize the computer equipment for additional clinical runs, training personnel,
and research.

The 1130 in most clinical laboratories is used for
recording patient laboratory data, collating, and formulating.
It produces printed summary reports from the stored information. At Yale, Dr. Seligson is working on an on-line data
acquisition system via paper tape at the Grace New Haven
Hospital using an IBM 1130 computer.

Current installations can be found at the University of
Pennsylvania, Philadelphia; Case Western Reserve, Cleveland,
Ohio, and Grace New Haven Hospital, Yale University, New
Haven, Connecticut; Uppsala University Hospital, Sweden,
and Spandau Hospital, Berlin, Germany (see Fig. 2).

Comments. The cost of the IBM 1130 is roughly
$2000 per month. The core storage capacity is 4096 or 8192
addressable binary words of 16 bits. This system can be
leased, rented, or purchased. The advantage of this system
is the feasibility of self-programming in FORTRAN or

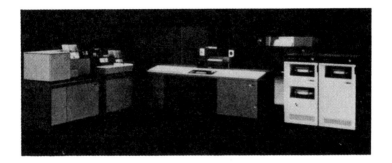

Fig. 2.   The IBM 1130 System with input-output devices.

assembly language.   The 15. 5-character-per-second selectric
typewriter and 300-per-minute card reader are the two most
common input media used.   This has a cartridge disc storage
capability with good reliability statistics.   The output unit is
an IBM line printer.   The 1130 is not, however, a multiprogramming computer.   One of the disadvantages of the 1130
is that there is no turnkey programming package available,
making a small data processing staff, including programmers
and analysts, mandatory.   This system has no special-purpose
terminals for remote input from the various laboratories and
is in most cases limited to card input.   Immediate access is
available at the console via a selectric typewriter.

C.   Berkeley Scientific Laboratory System

The BSL data processing approach to clinical laboratories consists of two systems, the Clin-Data and Chem-Data.
Each contains its own small computer, the PDP-8.   The Clin-
Data is intended to service manual input terminals and maintain
patient files through the use of a 500, 000-word disc file.   This

system can also be used to monitor the Technicon SMA/12 or
SMA/7A. If, however, the monitoring of a single- or dual-
channel autoanalyzer is desired in addition to the SMA/12 or
SMA/7A, it is necessary to add the Chem-Data System.

Patient information is entered into the Clin-Data by
teletype or card reader. The computer software directs the
preparation of work sheets and schedules which are then
returned to the test stations with specimens. Manual test
results are entered through BSL's own input terminal designed
for specific functions, e. g., hematology. Such numeric input
terminals will not accept alphabetic input.

Input terminals also may be interfaced with semiautomated test instruments. Operators visually verify results
before transmission. Completed test results are transmitted
on-line to the computer and patient files. For the automated
instrumentation, a work list is generated, which specifies the
order of the samples. It is also possible to use the special
purpose BSL terminals to enter automated test results into
the computer [14].

A typical installation might include five data input
consoles, one digital multiplexer with console controller, a
PDP-8 computer, a KRS-35 teletype-writer, two magnetic
tape drives with controller, and a Kleinschmidt printer.

Hospitals in which one or the other of the BSL systems
are located include: University of California in San Francisco;
Presbyterian-St. Luke's Hospital in Chicago; Clinical Research
Center of the National Institutes of Health in Bethesda, Mary-
land; St. Vincent's Hospital in Portland, Oregon; and the
U. S. P. H. S. Hospital in Baltimore, Maryland (see Fig. 3).

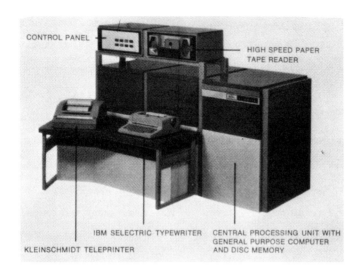

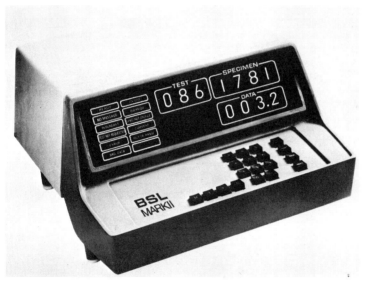

Fig. 3.   Berkeley Scientific Laboratories' Pathology
Clinical Laboratory Computer System and Clin-data Mark II
Terminal.

Comments. The cost of the Clin-Data System and the Chem-Data is roughly $145,000 (from $100,000 to $165,000). Lease charges for the two systems run approximately $3712 monthly for 5 years or $4350 monthly for 18 months; both figures include service charges [11].

An advantage in the BSL System is the special-purpose input terminals.

BSL provides a program package which initially includes options for minor modifications as may be desired, such as formating of the various outputs. The package will be supported and maintained if it is not changed. Should the laboratory need changes after the system is operational (which is usually inevitable) an additional charge is made under special contract. If the user makes his own changes, maintenance support on software is withdrawn.

BSL as well as Spear has had much trouble with the Kleinschmidt printer, which is down frequently enough to warrant a second printer as a backup. Those users who have gone to higher speed and more expensive printers have reported considerable improvement in service records.

A poor service record has been reported by users on the BSL terminals and the disc. One user has reported input terminal down-time of 20%. * Also, it should be noted that there is a need for linking the Clin-Data and Chem-Data into a unified chemistry and hematology system. This means that data from the two systems must be merged for a single patient-summary report.

D. IBM 1800 Control System

In this system the clinical laboratory instruments transmit results on-line to the computer in the general chemistry procedures. The 1800 then performs the functions of peak identification, validation of peaks (i.e., no bubble spikes or shoulders), prints error warnings if something has gone wrong, and updates patient records when valid results are available [9].

The 1800 processes the laboratory test requests by establishing two disc files: a patient file and a results file. The instrument worksheets are then printed. In addition, a form is usually printed that lists tests to be performed on each patient so that laboratory workers are aware when all of the patient's tests are completed. Laboratory worksheets for the off-line tests are also generated and the results from the various laboratories are merged into the final summary report at a later time. The typewriter, the 1092 Matrix keyboard, and the 2260 CRT are some of the possible terminals used for immediate data access.

In this system the main data entry is either via a matrix keyboard or a card reader/punch. The system also has a disc drive for storage, with up to two tape drives to be used as additional storage.

A precise worklist for each autoanalyzer is needed for specimen identification so that the technologist will know the order in which she must place serum cups on the sampler. This list is most important because the name of the patient is filed in the computer in this exact order to establish a one-to-one match. In some cases, the 1084 stub card reader with the T-40 sampler has been added for positive specimen identification (approximate cost $4500-$5000).

Laboratory instruments which have been interfaced to the 1800 computer include the Technicon AutoAnalyzers, the SMA 12/60, the Beckman DSA-560, the Coulter Counter, and the Coulter S Multiple-Channel Hematology System.

Hospitals which use the 1800 in the clinical pathology laboratory include: Houston Methodist Hospital in Texas; University of Colorado Medical Center in Denver, Colorado; St. Vincent's Hospital in New York City; University of Kentucky Medical Center in Lexington, Kentucky;* Johns Hopkins Hospital in Baltimore, Maryland; the Virginia Medical College Hospital in Richmond, Virginia; and Tubingen University Hospital in Tubingen, Germany (see Fig. 4).

Comments. The purchase cost of the 1800 system is approximately $200, 000-$250, 000; rental ranges from $4400 to $10000 per month and includes the peripheral equipment mentioned above [11]. To run an 1800 system a competent programming staff is necessary since only a limited software package is available. At present, IBM supplies peak-picking and file-structuring packages.

The 1800 has an efficient time-sharing executive program operating for the 16, 24, and 32K systems. Also, a multiprogramming executive program is available and operates on machines with core sizes ranging from 16 to 64K.

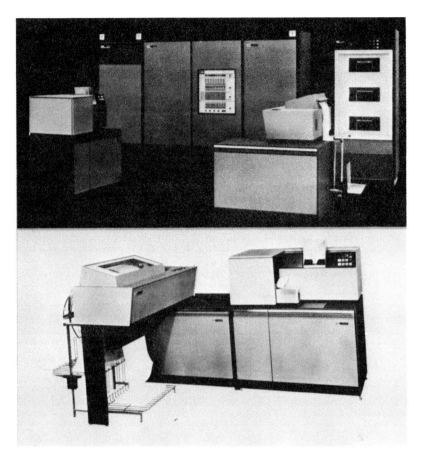

Fig. 4. IBM 1800 Data Acquisition and Control System
and IBM 1800 Input-Output Unit.

The 1800 system is usually too costly for the average

clinical laboratory. The system requires a good deal of

systems and customer engineers, as well as field engineering

support. The 1800 does not have a terminal system that can

be used in hematology, clinical microscopy, or bacteriology,

making its function mainly card oriented. Clinical chemistry,

however, is well served by this system.

E.   IBM 1080 Data Acquisition System

The IBM 1080 Data Acquisition System is designed to collect output signals from autoanalyzers and other laboratory instruments. It is an on-line data collection system but an off-line processing system. It records instrument readings and associated control data into punched cards or paper tape. As discussed above (Sipper Sampler Reader T-40), the system provides a solution to the problem of positive specimen identification. Once the cards are punched automatically by the 1080, they are taken to a general purpose computer for final processing and generation of reports under a software control procedure called Automatic Chemistry Program. The computers that can accept this program are the IBM System/360, 1440, and 1130.

A typical 1080 clinical laboratory data acquisition system consists of a 1081/Model 2 control unit, a 1057 (non-printing), or 1058 (printing), card punch, the 1084, and the 1082 card reader.

Hospitals in which the 1080 is in use include: Youngstown Hospital, Ohio; Lahey Clinic, Boston, Massachusetts; St. Francis Hospital, Wichita, Kansas; City Hospital, St. Louis, Missouri; Lakeland General Hospital, Tampa, Florida; University Hospitals, Boston; and the University of Tennessee Medical Center, Memphis, Tennessee (see Fig. 5).

Comments. The 1080 is not a computer; it is a highly sophisticated data collection system with the great advantage of including a superior specimen identification unit. The cost of the 1080 system is $600 per month. * The 1084 sample

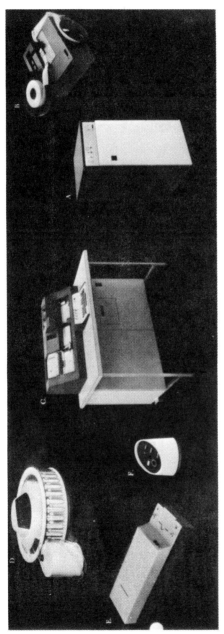

Fig. 5. IBM 1080 System, (A) 1081 Data Acquisition System Control; (B) 1055 Paper Tape Punch, Model 3; (C) 1057 Card Punch, Model 3; (D) 1084 Sampler Reader with the Technicon Sampler 40; (E) 1082 Card Reader; (F) 1083 Remote Control.

reader costs $3000 to purchase and the stub card reader,
$3600. In addition to the above hardware, it is necessary to
rent keypunch machines and employ operators. *

If a dedicated computer system is desired, the ACP
programs are adaptable to the IBM 1130. This computer can
be rented for approximately $2000 (or more) per month plus
programming cost and service. In most cases, however, the
1080 is used in the batch processing mode with the cooperation
of the hospital EDP Department. Immediate access capabilities are not available with this system.

The 1080 system works well provided there is effective
management. In more loosely organized laboratories the
system has been less successful. The IBM 1080 System
was actually withdrawn from the market in the fall of 1970.
The approach, however, is being picked up by other vendors
such as Info-Med in Princeton, New Jersey.

F. Digital Equipment Corporation

DEC offers the clinical pathologist the LINC-8 computer
and its successor, the PDP-12 (Programmed Data Processing).
The laboratory software available for these machines has
been the LABCOM-4 and 5 programs developed by Dr. Phillip
Hicks at the University of Wisconsin. These programs provide on-line monitoring capability for eight autoanalyzers for
the basic LINC-8 with peak picking and on-line quality control
checks of analytical instruments [5].

The only remote terminals used in this system are
teletypes which may be placed in peripheral laboratories.

Thus, information can be relayed directly to the patient's file via teletype keyboard. Summary reports, collection lists, and worksheets are printed on teletypes or line printers. The LABCOM software utilizes the cathode ray tube oscilloscope display at the console and has a keyboard which permits the user to specify the programs or data desired.

Dr. Hicks has recently developed a more extensive system than his original LABCOM-4. The Clini-Lab 12 uses LABCOM-5 software and has added a patient file system,* making possible a summary report previously not possible with LABCOM-4. A 300-line-per-minute printer is supported on this system.

The hardware configuration of DEC's Clini-Lab 12 is a PDP-12, with 8192 12-bit words of core memory, built in CRT display, A to D converter, and disc. The CPU is capable of servicing up to six teletype units in addition to the on-line interfaced laboratory instruments. The standard teletype is the only terminal provided on this system.

The LINC-8 system, used with LABCOM-4 programs, is present at: the University of Wisconsin Medical Center, Madison, Wisconsin; Mercy Hospital, Urbana, Illinois; BioScience Laboratory, Van Nuys, California; Ohio State University Hospital, Columbus, Ohio; Tershin Hospital, Tokyo, Japan; Duke University Medical School, Durham, North Carolina; Conemaugh Valley Hospital, Johnstown, Pennsylvania; and Union Hospital, Framingham, Massachusetts. At present, no laboratory is fully operational using LABCOM-5, however, the University of Wisconsin and Conemaugh Valley will most likely to be the first (see Fig. 6).

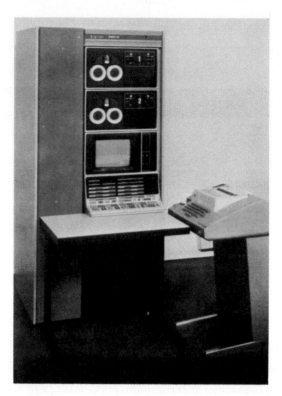

Fig. 6. Digital Equipment Corporation Clini-Lab 12
(clinical laboratory system using a PDP-12).

Comments. LINC-8, utilizing LABCOM-4, costs
approximately $98, 000 including disc, processor, 8K core
memory, five input teletype terminals, and a CRT at the CPU.
The system can be leased at $2802 monthly for 5 years with
service, or for $3452 monthly including a service contract
of $650 a month [11].

This system has an immediate access feature for
retrieving data. Output formats have been well received.
The teletype terminals, however, are slow and noisy. The

system has been employed principally in the chemistry section of clinical laboratories.

The cost of the Clini-Lab 12 system, utilizing LABCOM-5, is similar to other turnkey systems and falls into the $100, 000-$120, 000 purchase range. It is essentially a chemistry system. Also, as was true of the LABCOM-4, there are certain limitations to using teletypes as input or output devices at all areas of the laboratory.

The system of specimen identification employed in LABCOM-5 is somewhat different from other turnkey systems: here the technologist is solely responsible for the addition of the name of the patient to the specimen result after the run on the autoanalyzer has been completed. The advantage to this is that the trays can be loaded in any sequence. The technologist does, however, end up with additional work since it is up to her to identify the specimen as well as manually enter each identification by teletype in order to build her patient file.

LABCOM-5 software can be requested through DEC or Laboratory Computing, Inc. (Box 587, Madison, Wisconsin). The user must be aware of the fact that he is dealing with a two-party system in which one vendor is in charge of software and another of hardware. This leaves the laboratory in the position of middle man should there be an unresolved question as to whether hardware or software complications are keeping the laboratory from operating. *

G. Spear CLAS-300

The basic B-D Spear CLAS-300 System generally contains either 4000 or 8000 words of core storage and is

expandable to either 32,000 or 500,000 words, respectively,
of digital magnetic tape storage. The CLAS-300 features a
number of interesting characteristics for the clinical laboratory. The hardware system includes alphabetical-numeric
CRT displays and a typewriterlike keyboard. The central
CRT display can be used for graphic wave form presentation
from autoanalyzers and electrophoresis devices. The CRT
method of communication has proven to be fast, accurate, and
easily handled by the clinical laboratory staff, and is thus
proven to be one of the chief advantages of the CLAS-300
system [12].

The CLAS-300 system also includes a high-speed
multiplexor, an analog-to-digital convertor, and 12-28
channels for analog input data. Two 40-character-per-second
Kleinschmidt printers are included in the basic system.
Should a faster printer be needed, the computer can be interfaced to a 300-line-per-minute printing device. This system
provides on-line results from Bunker Ramo CRT entry stations.
The system also has immediate access capabilities for rapid
retrieval of information.

The CLAS-300 has been described as a turnkey system,
with B-D Spear providing a complete customized software
package for each installation. Current operating installations
can be found at the Moses Cone hospital, Greensboro, North
Carolina; Nassau Hospital, Mineola, New York; St. Joseph's
Hospital, Milwaukee, Wisconsin; Centralized Laboratory,
Long Island, New York; Central Pathology Laboratories,
Sacramento, California; University of Saskatoon, Saskatchewan,

Canada; and Perth Amboy General Hospital, New Jersey (see Fig. 7).

Comments. The CLAS-300 sells for approximately $75,000-$130,000, including two Kleinschmidt printers, 4K of core storage, 500,000 words of tape storage, and cathode ray tube and keyboard assemblies. The system can be rented for approximately $2500 monthly including maintenance.

The terminals allow two-way (I/O – input/output) communication to and from the CPU. The dialogue between the computer and technologist is via CRT terminal; the central terminal displays graphic wave form data allowing the technologist to use a light sensor to select fractional divisions, at which time the computer calculates the area under the curve for the divisions and produces a complete patient report. Other strip-chart wave forms can also be graphically presented on the CRT screen. Variable field length can be utilized for alphabetic data input using free English text. A good maintenance record is reported by B-D Spear users.

H. Infotronics

Infotronics Corporation of Houston, Texas, has installed its prototype clinical laboratory system at Clinical Laboratories, St. Louis, Missouri, under the direction of Dr. O. E. Hagebush. The system is designated as the 3055, which consists basically of a DEC PDP-8 CPU with teletype terminals and on-line single- and dual-channel monitoring in the chemistry area of the laboratory (see Fig. 8).

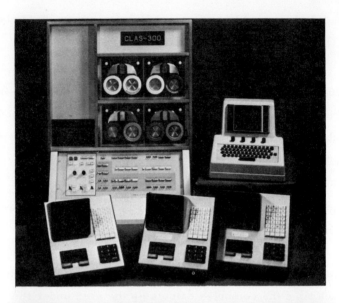

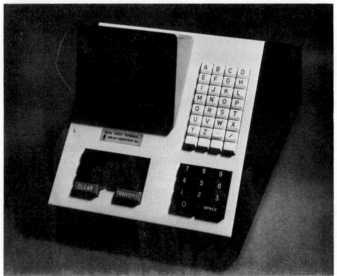

Fig. 7. Spear CLAS-300 System with terminals.

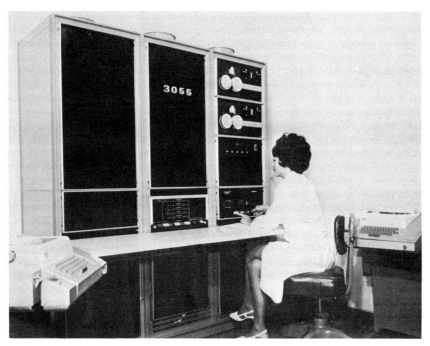

Fig. 8. Infotronics Custom 3055 System for automatic
data processing in clinical chemistry.

Comments. The cost of the 3055 is estimated at
$175,000 for purchase. At present, Clinical Laboratories in
Missouri is still the test site. The system gives reports on
individual tests for all chemistry tests. Hematology and
bacteriology are not included. The Infotronics system is,
therefore, dedicated to the chemistry area in the pathology
clinical laboratory. As in the DEC system, Infotronics has
no special-purpose terminals in the laboratory. Standard
teletypes are used for input and output of laboratory data.

I.   Diversified Numeric Applications

The basic DNA clinical pathology computing system includes a Raytheon 703 computer with 4-8K words of core and special purpose terminals built to DNA specifications.   The system has a 400-line-per-minute NCR printer, one teletype for input at the CPU, and one for output, which is located outside of the computer room.

The most unusual and unique feature of this system is its highly specialized special-purpose terminals — chemistry terminal, urinalysis terminal, and bacteriology terminal, all with the added feature of hard-copy verification capability at the terminal, as well as a special request/inquiry terminal. The system offers a turnkey software package with or without a card input system, as desired (see Fig. 9).

Comments.   The cost of the basic system is approximately $170,000.   The prototype has been installed at Hennipen County Hospital, Minneapolis, Minnesota.   Here a SMA 12/60 conducts peak picking on-line on a 28-second scan principle. Several single- and dual-channel autoanalyzers are added on-line to the system.   A second system is installed at the North Memorial Hospital, also in Minneapolis.

At the Hennipen installation, no card input capability exists, a factor that could cause special difficulty when the terminals or CPU are down.   The system is limited to a six-digit hospital number, a consideration not to be overlooked with the coming of the use of the social security number with nine digits.

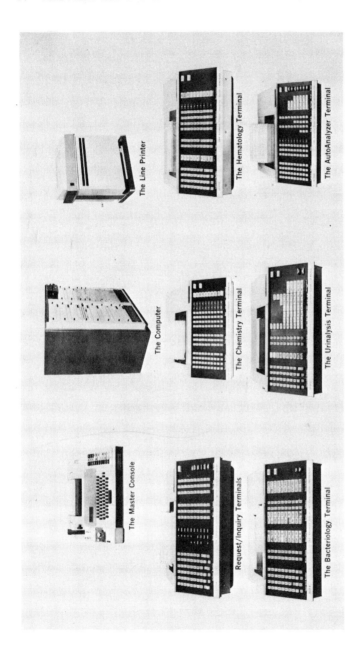

Fig. 9. The DNA Automated Clinical Laboratory System with special purpose terminals.

DNA emphasizes the importance of hard-copy verification, which is true. However, the counterpoint is made that the special-purpose terminals seem to be quite slow, (e. g., a 3-minute entry of bacteriology results for one person)* The system with its special terminals does not allow for free English text capability. The CPU can be queried via keyboard and the answer returned via hard copy on a teletype printout for immediate access purposes. For overall comparisons see Tables I and II.

IV. SUMMARY

In considering computerization in American pathology laboratories to date, we believe that competent management of the laboratory is crucial. Software and efficient direction of the computer system are more important than hardware considerations. Although hardware is indispensible, it is most unlikely that this aspect of the system will be slighted. However, integration of the computer system with laboratory operation, as well as adequate overall organization of the laboratory, may easily be neglected in planning.

Most computer vendors are eager to assure the potential buyer that their company can do the required job. Indeed, the unwary laboratory director may be forthrightly told that a given computer system is "perfect" for his pathology laboratory and then subsequently find that it is not adequate at all. We believe, then, that it is indispensable to compare various systems before computerization is undertaken and, secondly, that it is necessary to obtain competent opinions independent of the computer companies.

As a part of the planning involved in the installation of a computer system, it is desirable to outline and specify the daily and overall functions of the pathology laboratory: how many tests are to be run each day, contents of monthly reports, type of billing required, and retrieval of information desired. Only after the requirements of the laboratory have been specified will it be feasible to compare realistically the advantages and disadvantages of computer systems with regard to the needs of one's own laboratory [1].

We believe it is necessary for the pathology laboratory director to be personally committed to computerization if the system is to operate successfully. Responsibility for installing a computer system cannot be delegated to lower-level personnel or to a computer company. The entire laboratory must be efficiently organized and forcefully directed in order to arrive at effective computerization. Computer hardware is not a substitute for organization.

The concept of "turnkey systems" is often deceptive. The technical staff of the laboratory must become involved and supervision of the system has to be provided by the professional staff. This will usually require a high level of competency on the part of the professional staff. Furthermore, it is safe to predict that, at least in the beginning, computerization of the pathology laboratory will not reduce the technical staff and that it will be more costly than the prior procedure [8].

What are the advantages, then, of installing a computer system in the laboratory? First, and most important in our view, is the improvement in laboratory services which thus

becomes feasible. Test results can be more accurately and

rapidly obtained; this is particularly true if the laboratory

has a considerable workload. Related to the improvement in

clinical service is the fact that the successful installation of

a computer system will enable the laboratory to develop

capabilities not previously available. Among these are

immediate access to patient data and availability of computer

analysis for research.

REFERENCES

1. Association of Clinical Pathologists, Technical Methods Committee, Flynn, F. V., chairman, "Data Processing in Clinical Pathology," J. Clin. Path., 21, 231 (1968).

2. E. Cotlove, "Sample Identification for Automatic Data Acquisition," presented at the annual meeting of the Academic Clinical Laboratory, Physicians and Scientists, Yale-New Haven Medical Center, May 15-17, 1969.

3. P. R. Finley, F. Anderson, and R. Neese, "Electronic Data Processing in a Private Hospital Laboratory," Amer. J. Clin. Path., 48, 575 (1967).

4. W. Helmreich, "Sample Identification for Automated Analysis Systems," presented at the Technicon International Congress, Chicago, Illinois, June 4-6, 1969.

5. G. P. Hicks, M. M. Gieschen, W. V. Slack, and F. C. Larson, "Routine Use of a Small Digital Computer in the Clinical Laboratory," J. A. M. A., 196, 150 (1966).

6. A. Jahn, et al, "Mechanisierte Analysensysteme I Der Perkin-Elmer "C4" - Analysenautomat," Acta Medico-technica, 4, 105 (1970).

7. E. Kenzelmann, "Die Verwendung von Computern im Klinischchemischen Labor," (The use of computers in the clinical chemistry laboratory), Elektromedizin, 12, 140 (1969).

8. T. D. Kinney, and R. S. Melville, "Automation in Clinical Laboratories, " Lab. Invest., 805, 808 (1967).

9. J. Lukins, M. Ball, W. B. Stewart, N. Hill, and R. O'Desky, "Computerization in the Clinical Laboratory," presented at the spring meeting of COMMON, Chicago, Illinois, April 8-10, 1968.

10. M. V. Mathews, "Little Computers - Their Power and How to Make It Work For You, " presented at the annual meeting of the Academic Clinical Laboratory, Physicians and Scientists, Yale University, May 15-17, 1969.

11. Michigan Hospital, Computer Automated Pilot Project: Computer Automated Laboratory, a preliminary report, 1969, p. 35 (mimeographed).

12. H. C. Pribor, W. R. Kirkham, and R. S. Hoyt, "Small Computer Does a Big Job in This Hospital Laboratory, " Mod. Hosp., 110, 104 (1968).

13. A. E. Rappoport, W. D. Gennaro, and W. J. Constandse, "Should the Laboratory Have It's Own Computer?" Hosp. Progr., 50, 114 (1969).

14. S. A. Sondov, Clinical Chemistry Automation Using a PDP-8/L, Decus Proc., pp. 303-306, Spring, 1969.

15. J. V. Straumfjord, M. N. Spraberry, H. G. Biggs, and T. A. Note, "Electronic Data Processing System for Clinical Laboratories," Amer. J. Clin. Path., 47, 661-676 (1967); reprinted from Techn. Bull. Regist. Med. Techn., 37, 91 (1967).

16. M. Turoff, "Immediate Access and The User Revisited, " Datamation, 15, 65-67 (1969).

17. U.S. Senate, Judiciary Committee, "Medical Restraint of Trade Act, " hearings before subcommittee on antitrust and monopoly, 90th Congress, 1st session, Pursuant to S. Res. 26, on S. 260. U.S. Government Printing Office, 1967, pp. 315, 322, 337.

18. J. M. Walsh and S. A. Goldblatt, "A Punch-Card Laboratory Reporting System with a Cumulative Summary Format," J. A. M. A., 207, 1671 (1969).

9

Computer Applications in Acute Patient Care

Morton D. Schwartz
Associate Professor of Electrical Engineering
California State College, Long Beach, California

I. INTRODUCTION

The applications of computers and bioinstrumentation in intensive care units (ICU's) are just beginning. Many university medical centers (such as University of Alabama Medical School, Birmingham) have on-line requirements for patient monitoring or research, and a dozen or so hospitals, (such as Presbyterian Hospital, San Francisco) have data processing equipment for similar purposes. This chapter will try to provide insight into the different goals and requirements for the application of computers and bioinstrumentation systems within the intensive care units by presenting conceptual designs based on an extensive state-of-the-art review [1,2].

The system features will be applicable to the planning of ICU's [3] for teaching and research facilities. Most of the features are oriented toward the coronary and general ICU's; however, some features could be considered for burns, pulmonary, neurosurgery, and postcardiac surgery ICU's.

Some of the more significant design features are:

(1) Baseline System. Each patient unit is electrically
    wired so that when electronic instrumentation is
    brought to a bed the required slowly varying
    physiological parameters are monitored with
    alarms and displayed at the bedside and nursing
    station. The candidate parameters are ECG,
    heart or pulse rate, respiration rate, temperature,
    urine output, bed weight, and systolic, diastolic,
    and central venous pressures.

(2) System Option. Dynamic wave forms are obtained
    and sent by telephone line to a centralized compu-
    ting facility to give such derived parameters as
    cardiac output, pulmonary resistance and compli-
    ance, and nonelastic work per breath. Mobile
    equipment linked to the computer can be used for
    ECG diagnosis, pulmonary function tests, and
    diagnostic aids.

(3) System Option. Critical patient-care parameters
    are stored in the computer for report generation
    and teaching and research requirements. Storage
    oscilloscopes or TV monitors are used to display
    patient history data at the bedside and nursing
    station.

II. IMPLEMENTATION STAGES

It is advantageous to begin with a minimum monitoring
installation which may later be expanded by stages into a full

system. An implementation plan which will permit the achievement of the ultimate system in three phases is presented in Fig. 1 and discussed below. These stages are for illustrative convenience and are not meant to be arbitrarily restrictive. The implementation may start at any particular stage, or somewhere in between.

In stage 1, or the baseline system, a self-contained monitoring system is established. This system has the capabilities for monitoring the slowly varying physiological parameters and storing or reporting data on paper. Stage 2 then extends the system by using a data acquisition system and a portion of a centralized ADP system computer to store the slowly varying measured parameters in the patient's file so that reports, summaries, and trend analyses can be generated on the ADP terminal. (ADP is used to denote an automated data processing system which contains a computer for data collection and processing.) Stage 3, shown in Fig. 2, further extends this system by allowing high-frequency analog wave forms to be sent to the computer for filtering, processing, and/or storage. These wave forms can be regenerated or played back from the computer and shown on TV monitors at the bedside or nursing station in real-time. This ensures the physician or investigator that the data are being received and recorded properly by the computer. Furthermore, the TV monitors can be used for report generation, summaries, trend analyses, parameter graphical displays, teaching purposes, indicating alarms, and displaying derived parameters.

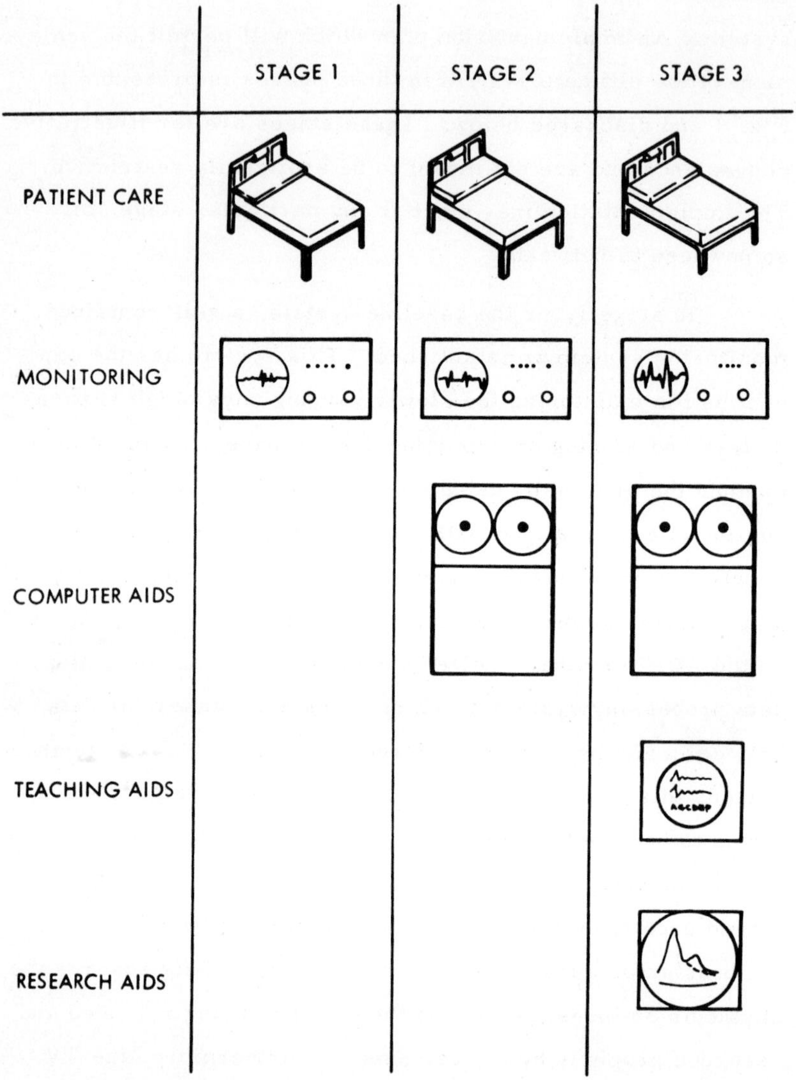

Fig. 1. Summary of monitoring system capabilities for
stages 1, 2, and 3.

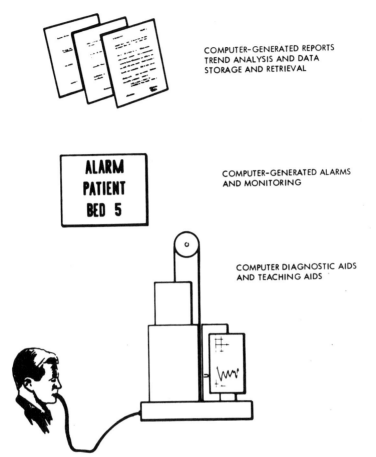

COMPUTER-GENERATED REPORTS
TREND ANALYSIS AND DATA
STORAGE AND RETRIEVAL

COMPUTER-GENERATED ALARMS
AND MONITORING

COMPUTER DIAGNOSTIC AIDS
AND TEACHING AIDS

Fig. 2. Stage 3 capabilities.

III. SYSTEM CONCEPTS

This section presents a conceptual patient monitoring
system which provides data connection terminals at each ICU
bed. These terminals would electrically connect every ICU
bed to its central nursing station to display and record critical
patient-care parameters. A patient monitoring equipment
pool is recommended for the sharing of instruments by all the
ICU's. However, this can be accomplished only if a single
set of instrument specifications are accepted, such as input/

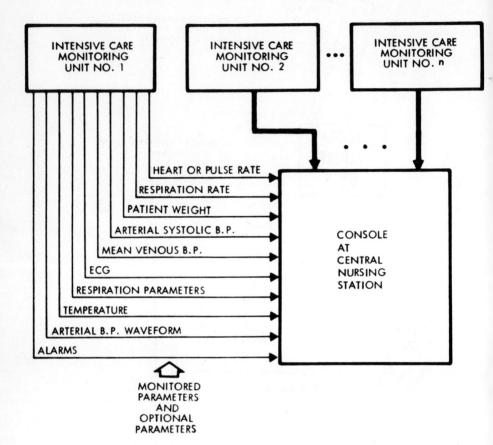

Fig. 3. Stage 1 intensive care monitoring system.

output characteristics, electrical connector configurations, and physical dimensions of the equipment.

A. System Capabilities

The monitoring system as shown in Figs. 3, 4, and 5 during stage 1 would have the following capabilities.

(1) Modular plug-in units on wall or cart for flexibility in monitoring physiological parameters.

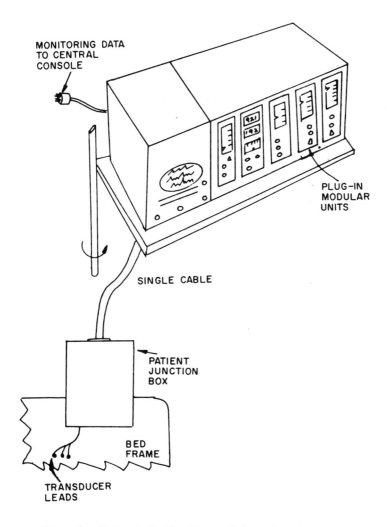

MONITORING DATA
TO CENTRAL
CONSOLE

PLUG-IN
MODULAR
UNITS

SINGLE CABLE

PATIENT
JUNCTION
BOX

BED
FRAME

TRANSDUCER
LEADS

Fig. 4. Swivel shelf with modular plug-in units.

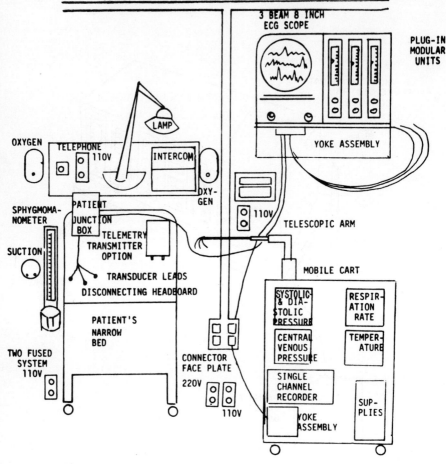

Fig. 5. Conceptual patient station with mobile cart.

(2) Alarms and displays at central console.

(3) Automatically monitor slowly changing physiological parameters or capture on trend recorders the following.

    (a) Heart and/or pulse rate.
    (b) Temperature
    (c) Respiration rate.
    (d) Systolic pressure.
    (e) Diastolic pressure.
    (f) Central venous pressure.

(4) Automatically capture on strip-chart recorders dynamic parameters such as the following.

(a) ECG.
(b) Pressure wave form.
(c) Respiration wave form.
(d) EEG.

(5) Measure parameters such as the following.

(a) Cardiac output.
(b) Blood gases, pH, and biochemical quantities.
(c) Respiratory gases.

(6) Automatically print patient monitoring record using electric typewriter at central console.

All instrumentation would be connected to the nursing station through an electrical conduit system with the following characteristics.

(1) Instrumentation on the swiveled shelf plugs into the shelf.

(2) The shelf has a single cable and plugs into the conduit system.

(3) Instrumentation on the mobile cart plugs into the cart.

(4) The cart has a single cable and plugs into the conduit system.

(5) Any unit of instrumentation can be plugged into any shelf or cart, and any cart can plug into the conduit system.

(6) All electrical transducers and electrical wires attached to the patient are plugged into the patient junction box.

(7) The patient junction box distributes the signals to the swiveled shelf and mobile cart through the conduit system.

The conceptual noncomputer monitoring system during stage 1 contains a readout device, such as an electric type-writer incorporated in the central nursing station, that provides visual sampled history of the slowly varying physio-logical parameters. Faster physiological phenomena such as ECG wave form, EEG, and respiratory wave forms can be observed on analog strip-chart recorders or oscilloscopes.

The physiological parameters such as systolic, dias-tolic, and central venous pressure, respiration rate, heart or pulse rate, ECG, and temperature will be sampled auto-matically on a regularly timed basis, depending on patient need. Under alarm conditions signals from the monitoring instruments will trigger the system into predetermined, higher sampling rates with coded identification of the patient initiating the alarm signal.

The special care unit would consist of a noncomputer monitoring system in which all of its beds are linked by an electrical conduit system to the nursing-station monitoring console. Up to six critical patient-care parameters, plus time, can be recorded per bed at the monitoring console's typewriter.

The typewriter format is easily separated into indivi-dual columnar records for the patient-history folder. Entries can be made into this columnar record by typing directly onto the paper record between rows of multipatient data. By using this media for secondary data logging, less information need be inserted into the ADP terminal in stages 2 and 3, thereby reducing the load on the information system. Slow-speed trend recorders would also be used to capture pertinent data in analog form. These data can then be reviewed for trends and placed in the patient file for later study. Slow-speed trend recorders are now under development that would allow 8 hours of patient data to be recorded on an 11-inch length of graph paper.

B. Instrumentation

The monitoring requirements for the special care units or ICU's were discussed above. A detailed discussion on some of the equipment required is presented here. The following modular plug-in equipment would be brought to any of the ICU beds if needed and placed on swiveled shelves as shown in Fig. 4.

    (1) Eight-inch oscilloscope to observe ECG and pressure wave forms (multibeam).

    (2) Heart-rate analog meter with ECG preamplifier.

The ECG, heart rate, and physiological wave forms would also be displayed at the central nursing station. An electric typewriter would print out all parameters being monitored and the bed number of the patient, and a trend recorder would capture the slowly varying analog wave forms. The patient junction box is used to concentrate all the transducer leads from the patient into a single cable which then connects the monitoring equipment on the swiveled shelf to the junction box. If the patient is moved, the junction box accompanies him to his new location and allows the patient to be quickly tied into the monitoring system through a single electrical cable.

Electronic monitoring of other physiological functions such as systolic and diastolic pressures, respiration rate, etc., would be required at certain times for patients in shock or with other complications and for teaching and research purposes. This monitoring equipment would have analog displays and would be placed on mobile carts next to the bedside. Using an electrical conduit system, this data as well as the ECG and heart-rate data would be brought to the central nursing station and observed on displays. Figure 5 shows a conceptual mobile cart with a telescopic arm. The cart would sit at the foot of the bed, and the telescopic arm would bring the leads from the foot of the bed over to the patient. Telemetry equipment might be employed as shown in Fig. 6 to monitor mobile patients or for research purposes. By locating the receiver on the swiveled shelf above the bed, the average distance between the patient wearing the transmitter and the receiver is minimized, thus producing a suitable signal-to-noise ratio.

There would be three sets of analog displays at the central nursing station for every 10 beds and one set of digital displays. The ECG and heart rate would be shown on the analog displays, and the slowly varying physiological parameters would be shown on the digital display and captured on trend recorders. The central nursing monitoring console would have the capabilities to: (1) sequentially cycle through all the designated beds and display the measured parameters or wave forms and parameter limits for each patient, (2) continuously display one to three beds without cycling, and

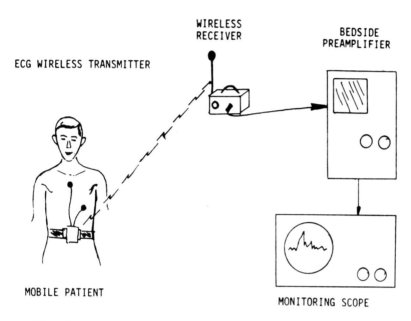

Fig. 6. Telemetry equipment to monitor mobile patients.

(3) automatically and immediately show the parameters under alarm whenever their limits are exceeded.

Every bed in the ICU would be tied into the electrical conduit system at the central nursing station. This should not imply that there is a full set of patient monitoring instru-mentation at every bed, but only that modular plug-in units can be brought to any ICU bed and tied into the electrical conduit system.

A full complement of patient monitoring equipment can not be kept at each ICU bed for economic reasons. Thus, a central monitoring equipment pool is proposed that would serve the ICU's. All the coronary-care beds would have bedside monitoring equipment, but other ICU beds would not. On the average, probably 20-40% of the ICU beds would have monitoring equipment.

The mobile monitoring carts can be similarly brought to any bed and tied into the electrical conduit system. The percentage of mobile carts would probably be 5-10% of the ICU beds.

C.   Central Monitoring Station

Examples of conceptual nursing-station monitoring consoles are shown in Figs. 7 and 8. Actually, the equipment would probably be located on several different counters with the time-elapsed meter and clock on the wall. The TV monitors and data phones or internal telephone lines would be installed during stage 3.

The computer-generated patient displays (reports and graphs) of parameters would be presented at the nursing console and, as desired, at the patient's bedside. A TV monitor or equivalent display system would be employed. Using TV monitors and an example, the system would operate as follows.

1. Nursing Console

Two TV monitors would be located at the nursing console. One monitor normally would sequentially present patient parameters, while the other would be used for particular displays such as an alarmed patient's parameters, a selected patient, trend warnings, required reports or graphs, etc. In the event of more than one emergency, it is likely

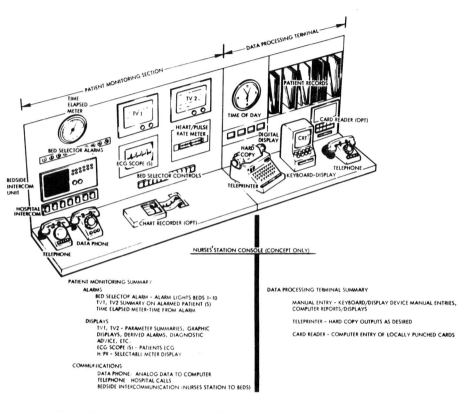

Fig. 7. Monitoring console at nursing station: example 1.

that the second TV monitor would stop its sequential scan and present information on the other alarmed patient. In addition, the means must be present to alert the staff if more than one alarm occurs at a time and the staff is concentrated in the area around the first patient under alarm.

2. Patient Station

The TV monitor at the bedside would be utilized to present selected parameters on that patient or, in the event

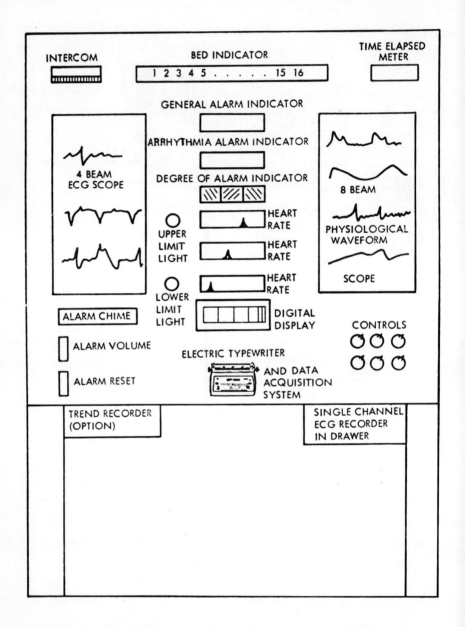

Fig. 8. Monitoring console at nursing station: example 2.

of an alarm, would provide a running list of the patient's parameters. Capability would exist for either numeric or analog graphic displays. Such displays at the bedside may have outstanding teaching potential. The type, frequency, and format of the displays could be altered by computer program changes.

Parameters that could be instrumented for automatic monitoring and entry into the computer include: room air temperature, skin temperature, rectal temperature, ECG, arterial pressure, airway flow, intraesophageal pressure, peripheral blood volume changes, and other parameters such as EEG. Along with these quantities automatically monitored, the following data can be obtained by manual or semiautomated techniques and introduced into the patient's computer data file: weight, blood gases, blood chemistries, and expired CO_2 and O_2. With all of these inputs, the computer-based system can report on a variety of parameters such as: patient number and time of report, systolic pressure, diastolic pressure, mean venous pressure, mean arterial pressure, heart rate, pulse rate, preventicular contractions, minute volume, tidal volume, respiration rate, alveolar ventilation, lung compliance, pulmonary resistance, work due to pulmonary resistance, O_2 uptake and CO_2 excretion, respiratory quotient, metabolic rate, temperatures, hematocrit, arterial pO_2, pCO_2, pH, and O_2 percent saturation, mixed venous pO_2, pCO_2, pH (catheterized patient), cardiac output, stroke volume, mean circulation time, peripheral resistance, and blood volume.

The intercom system could be used for special services such as blood gas lab, admissions, emergency, cafeteria, and for communication to the other ICU's. The bedside intercom would allow the staff at the bedside to communicate with personnel at the nursing station during emergencies, etc., and would allow the patients to signal or speak to the staff.

Analog displays on the console would be available for ECG and heart rate. However, there would be only three heart-rate displays for every 10 patients. The staff at the console can automatically or manually switch or cycle the analog displays through all beds as required. A digital display would give readings for up to six slowly varying physiological parameters and would be similarly cycled through the beds at specified time intervals. Under alarm conditions, the bed selector would indicate what bed has initiated the alarm, the typewriter would type in red the information indicating the bed in question, time, and up to six of the patient's slowly varying parameters, the analog displays would switch over and automatically monitor the patient, and the time elapsed meter would be turned on. If recorders are required, these would also be automatically turned on. "High" and "low" alarms are included on critical patient-care parameters. A trend recorder is considered as an option and has three multi-colored pens to give graphical summaries.

The characteristics of the console's operation are shown in Table I. There are three modes of operation: functioning under alarm due to arrhythmia or other reasons (general), switching bedside instruments to slaved console

TABLE I

Modes of System Operation

Console modules utilized in each mode of system operation	Modes of system operation at central monitoring console		2. Automatically or manually switch through beds	3. Continuously observe (lock on) 1 to 3 beds
	1. Alarm energized			
	Arrhythmia alarm	General alarm		
ECG scope showing lead II	x	x	x	x
ECG recorder turned on	x			
Trend recorder turned on				x
Heart-rate meter display	x	x	x	x
"High" limit heart-rate display	x	x	x	
"Low" limit-heart rate display	x	x	x	
Bed No. indicator	x	x	x	x
Time-elapsed meter	x			
Arrhythmia alarm indicator	x			
General alarm indicator (pressure, temp., respiration)		x		
Degree of alarm	x	x		
Physiological wave form scope (arterial pressure, etc.)	x	x	x	x
Alarm chime energized	x	x		
Data acquisition system	x	x	x	x

displays (manually or automatically), and continuously observing on the console's displays specific patients. For each
mode, the utilization of the console components is noted.

Under the switching mode, the three heart-rate meters
simultaneously present the upper alarm limit on the top display, the patient's heart rate on the middle display, and the
lower alarm limit on the bottom display for each patient.
This means that the upper and lower limits must be specified
for each patient and set into the console equipment. By
simultaneously displaying the limits and parameters, the
staff can quickly evaluate the significance of the observation.

If an alarm is energized at the bedside, the alarm
chime will be used and the "degree-of-alarm indicator" will
show by colored lights to what degree the parameter has
exceeded its limits in terms of standard deviations.

D.   Therapeutic and Emergency Equipment

Candidates for the therapeutic and emergency equipment are as follows.

(1)   External pacemakers which are used for temporary
pacing of the heart.

(2)   Defibrillators which are used for cardiac arrest
and serious arrhythmias.

(3)   Intermittent positive-pressure respirators which
are used for inhalation therapy.

(4)   Mechanical heart-massage apparatus and hand and
automatic mechanical resuscitators which are

used when closed-chest massage and resuscitation
are required.

(5) Automatic rotating tourniquets which are used for
treating congestive heart failure.

IV. DATA ACQUISITION CONCEPTS

This section presents the conceptual design for the
data acquisition system in the special care units for stages
1, 2, and 3.

A. Performance Characteristics – Stage 1

The performance characteristics of the conceptual
monitoring data acquisition system for stage 1 are listed in
Table II. This system provides for the monitoring of up to
six slowly varying physiological parameters per bed at the
central nursing station via a system which is sufficiently
flexible so that any bed can be instrumented as required.

Under alarm conditions a signal initiates an immediate
scanner sampling cycle and also causes the scanner to increase
its preset cycling rate so that the bed in question is examined
once every 2 minutes. Furthermore, a ribbon shift printout
on a typewriter is used to identify the patient under alarm,
and the bed selector indicates the patient. The scanner
continues to cycle until the patient's parameters return within
the allowable limits and the alarm circuit is manually reset
at the bed. All the instrumented ICU beds send analog signals
and alarms to the nursing station where they are observed on
trend recorders and displays and typewritten on paper.

TABLE II

Performance of Monitoring Data
Acquisition System: Stage I

---

1. Monitors up to six parameters per patient station

2. Prints out on one electric typewriter per central console

3. Prints out (if modules employed)

  - Identification number of bed being recorded
  - Time in hours and minutes
  - Heart or pulse rate
  - Temperature
  - Respiration rate
  - Systolic pressure
  - Diastolic pressure
  - Central venous pressure

  (No more than 30 patient parameters are monitored per
  central console)

4. Prints out format which is separated into individual
    columnar records for patient-history folder

5. Serves up to 12 patient stations per central console

6. Scans in various modes

  Normal scan — digital clock controls cycling rate of
    parameter sampler for normal and alarm conditions;
    15 minute to 8 hour cycle for normal; two-minute
    cycle for alarm

  Max scan — scanning occurs at the system's highest
    cycling rate

  Patient scan — scan only one patient station at maximum
    rate

  Alarm scan - alarm signal initiates an immediate
    scanner sampling cycle and causes a red ribbon shift
    on typewriter for patient identification

TABLE II (continued)

7. Indicates alarms

   In alarm scan, typewriter continues two-minute cycling
   until patient parameter returns within alarm limits
   and alarm circuit at the patient station is manually
   reset

   Each module at patient station has its own alarm indicator light with manually set alarm limits

   All module alarms are connected to patient bed selector
   alarm at central console

   If any patient parameter alarm is initated, alarm scan
   begins, patient bed selector alarm indicates bed
   number, and adjustable audible alarm is sounded at
   central console

   Patient parameters for bed producing alarm are viewed
   on numerical display (digital) by pushing button under
   lighted bed number on patient bed selector alarm

8. Displays digital readout on numerical display when

   Patient station number is selected on patient bed
   selector unit

   Automatic scan mode is selected on numerical display
   control

B. Data Acquisition System Elements

A list of the data acquisition components for stage 1
is shown in Table III. The data coupler controls the recording
operation of the typewriter. Push-button switches on the front
panel select the recording mode. In the normal scan mode,
the digital clock controls the cycling rate of the scanner for
normal and alarm conditions. When the data coupler "max-
scan-mode" switch is depressed, scanning occurs at the

TABLE III

Components of Data Acquisition
System: Stage I

---

1. Parameter sampler

   Scans multiple analog parameters and sequentially
   connects patient parameters to sample and hold unit
   of minicomputer

2. Sample and hold unit

   Provides analog to digital conversion of patient parameters at very slow rates

   Produces BCD output for typewriter and computer
   during stage 2 (can provide ASCII or EBCDIC codes)

   Displays digital readout on numerical display located
   on central console

3. Data coupler

   Interfaces between sample and hold unit and typewriter
   as well as computer in stage 2

4. Electric typewriter

   Automatically prints out patient data in columnar format

5. Digital clock

   Controls scanning rate

6. Patient bed alarm indicator

   Specifies which patient has exceeded alarm limits

7. Patient monitoring modules

   Amplifies transducer outputs for display and alarm
   checks

---

system's highest cycling rate. Finally, the alarm scan mode causes the system to scan the bed under alarm and type the measured parameters in red.

Normally, the beds would be periodically scanned only for teaching or research purposes so that the system would be activated only under alarm conditions. However, the system may assist the staff by automatically recording portions of the clinical record, monitor forms, fluid balance forms, and special graphic records at preselected times or as required.

The data coupler digital output for the slowly varying parameters is in the form called "binary coded decimal." This code or its equivalent is required in order to operate the typewriter and is used in the second stage to send the data to the central computer for storage, trend analysis, and computer-generated alarms.

The function of the parameter sampler or scanner is to accept multiple analog inputs and sequentially connect the signals to a single readout device. Normally a scanner can service 25 beds and be programmed by front panel push buttons to skip vacant beds. Under nonalarm conditions, the scanner in the second stage will service each bed at 2-minute intervals (or whatever is preselected on the digital clock) and will transmit the data to a computer. No typewritten printout will be generated unless requested.

Simplified diagrams of the system input instrumentation and output instruments are shown in Figs. 9 and 10. The latter diagram presents alternate candidate printout instruments in addition to the electric typewriter such as punched

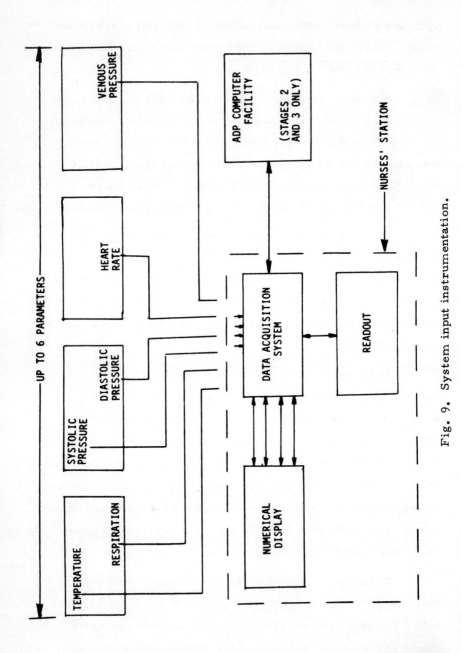

Fig. 9. System input instrumentation.

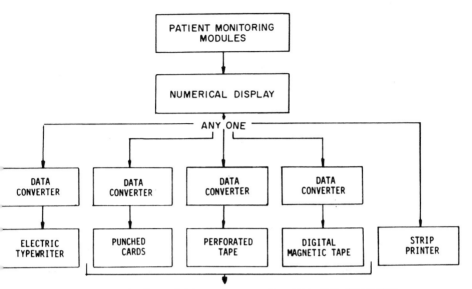

STRIP PRINTER CAN BE COMBINED WITH ANY OF THE 3 COMPUTER—
TYPE OUTPUTS FOR A PERMANENT VISUAL RECORD

Fig. 10. System output instruments.

cards, perforated tape, and digital magnetic tape. The data
coupler would have the capabilities for using any of these
output instruments, however, the special care unit would use
the typewriter in the baseline system with possible extension
to the other instruments, if required.

C. Extended System Capabilities

The stage-2 system incorporates all of the functions
and equipment involved in the first stage with the following
additions.

(1) Slowly varying digitized parameters would be sent
to the computer for time history recording, along
with trend and alarm testing.

(2) The ADP terminal at the nursing station would be used to display generated reports obtained from the patient data entered above.

The tie-in of the first stage to a computer to make a second stage system (computer-augmented ICU) was shown in Fig. 9. The slowly varying digitized parameters represent the output of the low-speed data acquisition system (sample and hold circuits). As in the first stage, up to six parameters are sampled per patient. These digitized parameters are serially transferred to the computer via telephone lines. Data transfer rates are in the order of 1.5-12 numeric characters per minute per patient, the higher rate being that of a patient in an alarm situation.

Using the ADP terminal, the computer-augmented system provides the following.

(1) Summary Reporting. Greater flexibility in obtaining summary reports (15 minutes, 1 hour, 8 hours, etc.).

(2) Prealarm Warnings. The computer can automatically monitor trends and provide warnings of impending alarms.

(3) Alarm Backup. In addition to the alarm capability built into the bedside analog modules, the computer can automatically check limits as a backup and report these to the ICU. Flexibility exists within the computer alarm program to set in different limits which vary the averaging time before alarming.

The stage-2 system does not impose stringent reliability requirements on the computer since it still continues to
operate as a stage-1 system in the event of computer down-
time. Patient records lost to the computer during this down-
time may be obtained later through manual entry from the
nursing console.

The conceptual stage-2 system is based on the assumption that a computer will be available and represents a computer-augmented patient monitoring system. This design
satisfies the baseline requirements and provides information
to assist the physician in the treatment of intensive care
patients. The system will automatically collect data, continuously monitor patients, anticipate critical trends, and display
data as required by the physician.

Sophisticated patient monitoring instrumentation has
been specifically developed to meet the need for patient data
collection. The ADP system can capture and coordinate these
data for optimum use by the physician and benefit to the patient.
It can anticipate critical trends before serious problems occur
and can be preconditioned to accept and store data, to calculate
averages, minimums and maximums and to alert the medical
staff when preset limits on slowly varying physiological parameters are exceeded. By storing critical patient signs, the
computer can be used for research and teaching purposes.

When critical trends are reported, the staff could take
corrective action prior to the emergency. In this way it may
be possible to concentrate on a particularly distressed patient
during emergency conditions without compromising the attention

due other patients since their data would be collected, compared to safe limits, trends predicted, and stored for subsequent review.

The ADP system could also assist in many of the
routine nursing tasks such as charting and record keeping.
The exact duties of the digital computer can be altered readily
by changing the software or programming. In this way the
system is flexible and can be adjusted to meet the changing
intensive care needs.

From the nursing station the physician can call for
an in-depth review of data that may influence the diagnosis or
treatment of the patient.   The display of data and reports are
presented at the bedside or nursing station.   The physician
calls for this display of data by executing a few typewritten
statements on the hospital data processing terminal.

Critical patient-care parameters are monitored with
alarm under local control at the nursing station. Data storage
and trend analysis are provided by the ADP system. In addition, the ADP system can also check for alarms as requested.
Data and critical patient-care parameters are initially stored
on the computer disk and then automatically accessed and
processed according to techniques which have been previously
defined by the medical staff and programmed into the computer.

An example of patient data processing is shown in
Fig. 11. Steps 1, 2, 3, and 4 collect and store patient data.
Steps 5 and 6 perform a limit check to detect readings which
are out of limit according to values which have been previously
established by the attending physician. Step 6 reviews previous

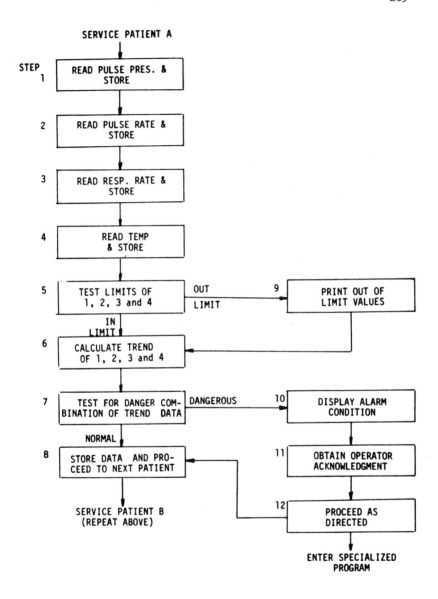

Fig. 11. Patient monitoring program.

data and predicts what data readings are expected at future
time intervals of interest. Step 7 performs a test that uses
these predictive readings. Thus, a dangerous combination
may be detected before it actually occurs. The staff would be
immediately alerted that a critical combination is expected
and a "fail-safe" staff acknowledgment is required by the
computer program. After a warning, step 10 is acknowledged,
and the program can be directed to display critical patient
signs for the physician or return to the servicing of other
patients.

The ADP system can provide the following services
to the ICU.

(1) Storage of critical patient-care parameters.

(2) Evaluation of selected data for trend analysis.

(3) Assistance in charting and report generation.

(4) Computational support for teaching and research.

(5) Establishment of rapid communication with special
hospital service areas.

(6) Allocation of personnel and resources available to
the ICU.

D. Data Capture

In the conceptual system, medical record data, such
as clinical observations and events occurring at the bedside,
are manually entered into the ADP system at the ADP terminal
located within the nursing station. Prepunched cards, mark-
sensed cards, or typewriter inputs may be used to allow the
ICU staff to enter data in a sequence acceptable for computer
processing and without the need for coding. Repetitive data,

such as regularly scheduled medications and dosages, may be entered automatically by inserting prepunched cards which contain all the information, including name of drug, dosage, and route of administration. Critical patient-care parameters which are monitored would be automatically entered into the ADP system.

The data most acceptable for computer processing are the monitored critical patient-care parameters which are stored and checked for alarms and trends and the medical record data such as the following.

(1) Medications.

(2) Liquid and solid intake and excreta.

(3) Physical data such as height, weight, and position of patient.

(4) Clinical observations such as signs and symptoms.

(5) Critical patient-care parameters which are not automatically sent to computer and are measured at discrete time intervals such as cardiac output, end tidal alveolar CO_2 concentration, and oxygen consumption.

The total number of medical record data entries per ICU patients can range from 10-75 records for an 8-hour shift with each record containing from 50-120 alphabetical and numerical characters. In addition, the monitored data can range from 1.5-12 numerical characters per minute for slowly varying physiological parameters, and 800-8000 numerical characters per second during stage 3 when high-frequency analog wave forms are digitally stored in the computer. Since

the medical staff is on-line with the computer, automatic
editing and correction of the entered data are possible. Immediate filing and on-line retrieval are also possible.

The ADP system can generate on-line preparation of
chronological listing of all entries made over a specified time
interval when requested. Under normal conditions these
reports are prepared on a batch basis at the end of each
nursing shift and at the end of a 24-hour period. Furthermore,
summary reports can be prepared that contain averages and
standard deviations of the digital values of the vital signs,
totals of volumes of intake and output, and a list of medications
administered that indicates the doses and the starting date for
each. Graphic plotting of critical patient-care parameters
can be achieved automatically at the central ADP facility or
on the ADP terminal at the nursing station by means of a
plotter connected on-line, CRT displays, or by use of an electric typewriter to emulate a plotter. These plots can be
prepared on a variable time axis so that trends and fluctuations
of vital signs over short or long periods of time can be visual-
ized.

E.   Final System

The stage-3 system represents an extension of the
stage-2 system in the following performance capabilities.

(1) <u>Dynamic Data Analysis.</u> The system provides
capability to record and analyze dynamic patient
parameters through the tie-in of higher bandwidth
analog data to the ADP center. More sophisticated

research and diagnostic analysis may be performed
such as ECG analysis, pressure wave form analysis,
arrhythmia studies, etc.

(2) Derived Parameters. The capability to obtain
secondary or derived parameters is increased.

(3) Patient Displays. The incorporation of TV or
other display devices allows for the nursing station
and patient bedside display of any computer-generated report including numeric and graphic displays.
The type, format, and frequency of the display
would be flexible in that changes would be incorporated by computer program (software) changes.

(4) Calculations. In addition to derived parameters,
it appears reasonable that the stage-3 system
would extend the ability to perform calculations
both from manually entered parameters and from
special test data automatically fed to the data
acquisition system.

(5) Training Aids. Training aids are required in all
the stages of the special care system development.
Simulation units would be set up to validate system
concepts and would also be used for training purposes. Stage 3 adds considerable capability for
the ICU in the area of training aids. First, the
ability to store and play back from the computer
either analog or digital stored information allows
for utilization of the operating system for training
and teaching either at the ICU console or at a

special training console. Secondly, computer-
generated displays would be easily sent on to a
special training console. The concept of play back
of trend warnings followed by an alarm could be
utilized. These aids could be developed by recording situations of interest and/or the employment
of simulated situations.

(6) System Self-Check. As operational experience is
obtained and as the clinical use of the computer as
a tool is increased, consideration can be given to
automating related support system functions such
as automatic checkout of the system to isolate
malfunctions, automatic or semiautomatic calibration of instruments, etc.

The equipment components added by the stage-3
system are as follows.

(1) Computer-generated displays (TV or equivalent)
at nursing-station console and patient bedside.

(2) Communication equipment – telephone lines,
sending-receiving amplifiers, and switching
circuits to handle the higher bandwidth analog
lines.

(3) ADP center equipment.
  (a) Communication equipment.
  (b) Data acquisition system.
  (c) Data recording system.
  (d) TV cameras or equivalent for transmitting
       computer-generated reports to ICU.

REFERENCES

1. M. D. Schwartz, "Computers and Bio-instrumentation in Intensive Care Units," Proc. 5th Rocky Mountain Bio-engineering Symposium, pp. 93-97, 1968.

2. M. D. Schwartz, "Design Features for Intensive Care Units," Proc. 20th Annual Conference on Engineering in Medicine and Biology, p. 30-6, 1967.

3. M. D. Schwartz, "Planning Patient Monitoring Systems," Proc. 8th International Conference on Engineering in Medicine and Biology, p. 17-12, 1969.

10

A Computer Based Information System
for Patient Care

Homer R. Warner
Department of Biophysics and Bioengineering
University of Utah and Latter Day Saints Hospital
Salt Lake City, Utah

I. INTRODUCTION

Since June, 1964, a Control Data 3200 computer
system has been installed in the Latter Day Saints Hospital in
Salt Lake City, Utah. This system in its inception was used
to develop research programs and time-sharing software for
use by the medical community in the Salt Lake City area. As
a result, a software and hardware system called MEDLAB
has been developed [1, 2]. Using this system, research

---

*Portions of this chapter have been adapted from the following
articles: "Computer System for Research and Clinical
Application to Medicine, " by T. Allan Pryor, Reed M.
Gardner and W. Clinton Day, published in AFIPS-Conference
Proceedings, 33, 1968; "Experiences with Computer-Based
Patient Monitoring, " by Homer R. Warner, published in
Anesthesia and Analgesia, 47, No. 5, Sept.-Oct. 1968; and,
"A 'Link Trainer' for the Coronary Care Unit, " by Homer
R. Warner and Albert Budkin, published in Computers and
Biomedical Research, 2, No. 2, Oct. 1968, and reproduced
by permission of the publishers.

programs were developed for cardiovascular studies. It
soon became apparent that the programs which were being
developed could also be used in a clinical environment. In
recent years, as the computer system was expanded, clinical
application became increasingly important. At the present
time the system is used in a variety of ways, including admission screening, maintenance of patient records, patient
monitoring in intensive care units, and training of coronary-
care nurses. This chapter presents the major hardware and
software features of the system and describes the major areas
of clinical application.

II   HARDWARE CONFIGURATION

The system used for both research and clinical applications is made up of three computers located at the L. D. S.
Hospital. A block diagram of the system is shown in Fig. 1
which shows the two computers – a CDC 3200 and 3300, the
3200 being used for research and program debugging and the
3300 being used strictly for operational clinical applications:
the small Digital Equipment Corporation PDP-8/S computer
is used as a teletype buffer driver to provide hard copy at
distant hospital sites. Although the 3300 has expansion capabilities which the 3200 does not have such as paging memory,
memory protect, etc. , the 3300 used has essentially the
same capability as the 3200 computer. Therefore, both
machines are hardware and software compatible and communicate through common disc units.

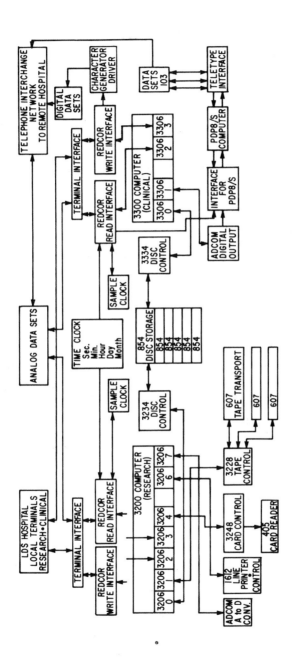

Fig. 1. System block diagram

There are three pieces of equipment identical on each machine which are critical for hardware and software interchangeability (listed as follows).

(1) The disc storage units.

(2) The REDCOR Corporation read and write interfaces, which are the adapters for communicating with the remote terminals and the handling of the physiological signals coming either from a patient or an experimental set up. The read interfaces for both machines are identical and analog signals are presented in parallel to the analog multiplexers of both interfaces. Thus, a program can be debugged, checked out and made operational on the 3200 research system with no change of channels or program. If the analog-to-digital (A-to-D) converter or computer system for the clinical system fails, the clinical operating system can be transferred to the 3200 machine with a minimum of rewiring (approximately 10 minutes required for changeover after the problem is diagnosed) and the assurance that the analog signals will be correct.

(3) The write interfaces on both machines are identical and are connected such that they can be transferred from one machine to the other with a minimum of difficulty (approximately 10 minutes).

The two machines are different in their hardware configurations since the 3200 is used for program compilation, printing, and magnetic tape capability for program and data storage. The extra peripheral equipment on the research machine includes a 1000-card-per-minute card reader, a 1000-line-per-minute printer, three high-speed magnetic tapes, and one special-purpose high-speed A-to-D converter. The 3300, or clinical machine, on the other hand, has a special output interface for the small PDP-8/S computer used to drive teletypes at the remote sites for hard-copy reporting of clinical and experimental information. Both machines are capable of operating remote terminals both from sites within the hospital and remote sites at other hospitals, experimental laboratories, and clinics.

1. Remote Terminals

Figure 2 shows a photograph of a typical remote terminal through which an experimenter communicates with the computer [3]. This remote terminal consists of a Tektronix 601 memory display unit, control and timing circuits for operation of this display unit, a decimal keyboard, and two 12-bit octal thumbwheel switches for coding information into the computer. Also shown on the front panel are indicator lights which tell the operator the state of the computer, the state of his program, and various other indications.

In a typical operation, the user calls a program by dialing a code into the octal switches, then presses the CALL button which interrupts the computer. The computer reads the octal switch and displays instructions back to the operator on the face of the memory display unit. The display unit is

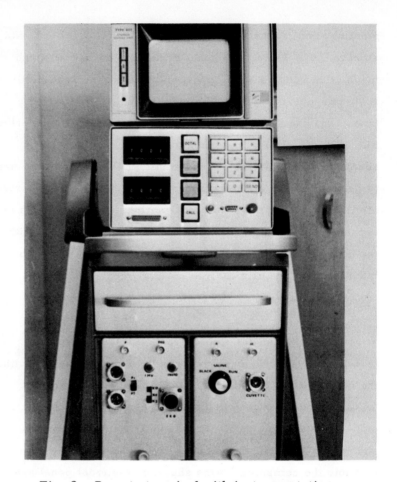

Fig. 2. Remote terminal with instrumentation.

capable of displaying 400 characters in a 25-column by 16-row
pattern or graphical information with a capability of 512 horizontal and 512 vertical dots.   In addition to its capacity as a
remote computer display terminal, the terminal can also be
used as a conventional three-channel memory oscilloscope by

pressing a push-button switch on the front panel. This feature allows the operator to quickly check signal-level qualities to be presented to the computer and insure that they are within range of the A-to-D converter and of adequate quality for the desired computer analysis. The display will revert from a conventional oscilloscope to a computer display terminal upon receiving an erase pulse from the computer, thus assuring that no computer-generated information is lost while the operator is viewing wave forms.

The processing of analog signals is presently carried out independent of the display terminal. As a standard package, each laboratory or clinical area is assigned three analog channels. These three channels are used for multiple purposes. For example, the three channels could be carrying pressure information, electrocardiographic information, densitometry information, etc., depending on the requirement of the user. This three-channel requirement was primarily determined by an electrocardiographic analysis program where three simultaneous lead signals are necessary. A second reason for making three analog channels a standard configuration is that three-channel data sets for telecommunication to distant sites are available for processing of data from remote hospitals.

The remote terminals with instrumentation can be constructed for a cost of about $3000; a character generator added for operation of remote sites costs an additional $1200. With the capability of both alphanumeric and graphical functions, this terminal becomes an extremely flexible convenient module for use in both clinical and experimental applications.

Since most of the physiologic signals are analog, it
was necessary to develop extensive front-end signal condi-
tioning equipment for the computer operation. An objective
in the development of the front-end equipment was to provide
extremely stable, highly reliable instrumentation, such that
a person with a minimum of instruction and training could use
it. The lower part of Fig. 2 shows the front panel of a typical
instrumentation package. Note that there are no control knobs
for adjusting gain or bias of the analog signals from the transducers and that there are a minimum number of control
switches for operator use.

The analog front-end system is made up primarily of
integrated-circuit operational amplifiers, with all signals
being amplified from their low-level condition to a high-level
($\pm$ 10 volts) condition for transmission to the computer, either
over hardwire connection or a telecommunication link. In
each case, signals are conditioned for optimum use by the
computer and by the telecommunication link by amplifying and
adjusting the offset for full-scale capability of computer and
communication link.

Experience has shown that minimizing the number of
controls and adjustments makes the system easier to use,
both by experienced and nonexperienced operators, and also
increases the confidence of the operating personnel. As a
typical example of an instrumentation application where this
type of approach has been used, consider the pressure transducer amplifier which amplifies signals from a balanced
Wheatstone-bridge strain gage. The gage itself can be

balanced, the amplifier or amplifiers could each have a separate offset control, the gage excitation could be varied, the amplifier gain could be varied, and so on. To minimize the problems in setup of a pressure transducer, only one control is provided and is made an integral part of the transducer system. The excitation voltage on the gage is fixed, the sensitivity of all the strain gages have been calibrated to a standard level and all pressure amplifiers are set up with the standard gains. A fixed offset has been programmed into the amplifying system and the only adjustment that need be made by the user is gage balance which compensates for varying fluid levels of the patient. Therefore, a pressure system which is usually complicated and difficult to handle becomes a simple set up procedure which a nurse or inexperienced technician can adequately handle and get results that are technically adequate and, in fact, as good as an experienced operator can obtain.

As can be seen from the foregoing discussion, the computer system has been designed with both a research investigator and a clinical investigator in mind, with standard packages designed and constructed which aid both. The system is also easily adaptable to special-purpose experimentation with signal levels that can be conditioned with a great amount of flexibility for the occasional user who has special requirements for signal levels, sampling rates, and timing.

Operation of terminals from remote hospitals is made over voice-grade direct-distance dial compatible telephone communication link. As far as the user is concerned, operation from a remote hospital is essentially the same as operating a local terminal.

The basic remote terminal, which is not much larger than the 201 data set (Fig. 2), is completely transportable and can be taken anywhere telephone communication facilities are available and used to communicate with the MEDLAB system. Applications for stand-alone communication terminals of this type are expected in tumor registry programs, radiation treatment planning, and other areas where analog signals are not necessary. When analog signals are required, Bell System data sets 604A and 604B, an analog transmitter and receiver, respectively, are used to send three channels of analog information simultaneously. The analog data bandwidth of these FM multiplexed channels is dc to 100 cycles for each channel. Cross-talk and signal-to-noise characteristics and bandwidth of these channels is adequate for transmission of most clinical physiologic information. The requirements for three channels are dictated by the vectorcardiographic system which requires three simultaneous channels of ECG. With a slight modification of this system it is possible to use a touch-tone telephone keyboard and a 604A/B, 401J data set configuration to transmit electrocardiograms and other physiologic data from any patient room within a hospital by installing phone jacks in the rooms and using the internal television distribution system of the hospital to transmit instructions and results to the operator on the television receiver located in the patient room.

A "program-line" connection is operational between the neurophysiology research laboratory at a remote hospital.

This type line is one which is commonly used by FM music stations and is conditioned to have "flat" frequency response from 50 Hz to 8 kHz making it ideally suited for transmission of action potentials.

Presently, there are systems in four hospitals using the communications terminals and one additional hospital using a hardwire connection. Plans call for region-wide screening clinics to be conducted by state, local, and private health organizations. With these terminals, health services can be provided to remote communities that heretofore were available only to patients at major hospitals.

III. SOFTWARE CONFIGURATION: THE MEDLAB SYSTEM

Design of a system for servicing physiologic needs presents some interesting problems. Computing speed is essential to accomplish certain tasks, and yet, on the other hand, some physiologic events occur very slowly compared to the computing time required to keep up with them. Thus, if the user is to have the computer when he needs it for this kind of work, it is necessary that a system be devised for rapid switching among programs. Such a time-sharing scheme has among programs. Such a scheme, called time-sharing, has been implemented on the Control Data 3200 at the Latter Day Saints Hospital in Salt Lake City.

A.   The Time-Sharing Monitor

The time-sharing monitor, called MEDLAB [2], resides in the memory of the central computer which, in turn, communicates with a variety of peripheral devices. Programs

or instructions are entered into the computer initially through
a card reader and are then stored on magnetic discs from
which they can be called into memory from any of the remote
stations. Data on patients in the hospital are also stored on
magnetic discs for ready access. When a patient is discharged,
his record is copied onto a library tape, where it is stored
permanently. Program listings and reports are generated on
a high-speed printer at the rate of 1000 lines per minute.

The analog-to-digital and digital-to-analog conversion
system forms the basic link to the remote stations. Presently,
there are 19 remote stations in five different hospitals attached
to our system. To each of these users operating from his
remote station, the computer appears to be under his command
and he can operate essentially independently of other users on
the system.

The 32,000 words of core memory are allocated as
follows to accommodate multiprogramming: in the top 5000
words of memory is the monitor program, which contains not
only the instructions that control switching among the programs
in memory, swapping of programs in and out of memory, and
sampling of data, but also a set of reentrant subroutines which
can be used by any of the user programs to accomplish such
tasks as writing on the oscilloscope, converting numbers
from binary to decimal, and inserting answers into messages.
This latter function considerably reduces the programming
the user must do to accomplish his goals.

From four to six real-time programs (up to 2000
words in length for any one overlay), which are actively

sampling data, may be in memory at any one time, and programs not sampling may be swapped onto discs temporarily
while other programs are being run. The lower part of core
memory is reserved for compilation and assembly of new
programs and execution of FORTRAN programs, which may
or may not communicate with the real world through one of
the remote stations. Those that do communicate with the
real world carry a higher priority than those that do not, in
the sequence in which jobs are executed. The organization of
data on the magnetic discs, whether from experimental ani-
mals or patients, follows a common format.

B. Differences Between the Research and Clinical Systems

The software available on the 3200 (research) system
and that on the 3300 (clinical) system are quite similar, but
some important differences exist. A major difference is the
type of program which can be run under either system. On
the 3300 system, which is used for clinical applications, there
are 12 partitions within core memory, each partition being
approximately 2000 words in length. Only those programs
which are designated clinical real-time programs and have
been written in assembly language are allowed to run within
any of the 12 partitions. Since the user can have only 2000
words of core at any time, most programs are written as a
series of overlays to be read in as needed into the same
partition. These programs must have reached a high degree
of reliability before being allowed to run on the clinical
system. The clinical executive monitor contains a dictionary
of the programs allowed, and if a program is not in that

dictionary a message is written on the display unit at the
terminal indicating that the program is not allowed. No
debugging of programs is allowed on the clinical system. All
debugging must be performed on the research system.

Software-wise there is no interaction between the
research system and the clinical system. The research
system is unaware of whether the data generated on any disc
is generated by a program being run on the research or the
clinical system. All data which are generated by either
machine and stored on disc are accessible by the research
system for report generation on the line printer.

C. Compilation of Data

This file organization is designed to provide for addition of new types of information in the future and still maintain a basic format, so that the same search, edit, and
analysis programs can be shared by a wide variety of users.
At the start of each file is a count which keeps track of how
many entries are currently in the file and where the next
word of data is to be stored. Entry of a field of data is
preceded and ended by a code which uniquely defines the kind
of data and the number of data words in the field. The second
word is the time and date, read automatically by the computer
from an external clock when the entry is made. Thus, any
user may define a new field of any length and add it to this
file.

D. Examples of Data Code

A general program has been written for introducing a
variety of physiologic measurements into the computer, which

is now in use in several diagnostic heart-catheterization laboratories connected to our system. This permits the user to initialize a file on a patient and call a variety of subprograms to analyze data in any sequence. To do this, a four-digit rotary switch on the remote console is used. The first digit indicates the type of analysis to be performed. For instance, 0 is an oxygen-saturation measurement, 1 is a pressure wave, 2 is a dye curve, and so forth. The second digit indicates the state of the patient. For instance, 0 means the patient is at rest, breathing room air, 3 means the patient is breathing oxygen during exercise, and so forth. The last two digits are used to indicate the position of the catheter tip in the circulation.

The operator dials the desired code and presses the interrupt. The code is interpreted by the computer and this interpretation is presented back on the oscilloscope for confirmation by the operator. If one or more of the digits was in error, the code is redialed and sent again. Until the same code is sent twice, the program will not proceed. When the data are on the line (for instance, the pressure to be measured appears free of artifact) the interrupt is pressed once again, and the analysis begins. The results are displayed back immediately to the operator, who may choose to discard the data or save them by writing them on the disc to be included in a later report.

Figure 3 shows the presentation made on the oscilloscope to the operator on completion of analysis of an indicator-dilution curve. At the bottom is the recorded curve plotted back as milligrams per liter and superimposed on this, the

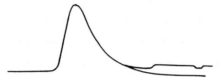

Fig. 3. Information displayed to operator within 1 second after completion of sampling following injection of indocyanine green dye.

experimental extrapolation carried out by the computer, so that the operator has some means for evaluating the adequacy of the analysis.

At the top are the calculated values: cardiac output is 4.16 L./minute. "M. I." is the mitral insufficiency index, which should be 1 or greater in a normal subject, and measures the skewness of the curve; this is a useful empiric index for the presence of mitral insufficiency in the absence of a left-to-right shunt. Next are shown appearance time, buildup time, mean circulation time, and central blood volume. At any time during the procedure and at the end of the procedure the operator may review and edit the data accumulated on the disc.

Figure 4 shows one page of data presented on the face of the oscilloscope. The "1" on the first line indicates that the patient is exercising and an oxygen saturation reading of 101 was obtained with the catheter tip in the "wedge" position.

```
1 W E      101
1 P.T      52/ 26    39
1 R V      84/ 15    20
2 R D      100
0 R D      97/ 64    77
0 R D        93
0 C . 0 .          4.16
  M . I .          1. 1
  A . T .        12.25
  B . T .         4.75
  M . C .        20. 0
  C . V .         1.38
```

Fig. 4. One page of data displayed during edit routine.

The next reading is a measurement of pressure in the pulmonary trunk, with the systolic, diastolic, and mean pressures shown. At the bottom is a cardiac output measurement by the dye method.

Pressing a zero causes the next page of data to be presented on the oscilloscope. Values may be deleted or altered by the operator, who may request any number of copies of a printed report upon completion of his editing, including a computer-generated summary of the abnormalities present. Thus, before the catheter is removed from the circulation, the data are completely analyzed, and if any question exists about the significance of some of the data, repeat measurements can readily be made. A direct extension of these techniques is their application in the operating room and at the bedside.

IV. APPLICATIONS TO PRE- AND POSTSURGICAL MONITORING

On the afternoon before surgery, the patient is taken to a special laboratory equipped with a remote computer station, where a tiny central aortic pressure catheter is introduced by

a technician.   Using a special armboard* which is floor mounted
and can be positioned next to any type of bed or table, the
patient's wrist is extended and local anesthetic is introduced
around the radial artery.   Then a thin-walled 18-gauge needle,
connected by a special catheter assembly+ to a strain-gauge
manometer, is introduced into the artery percutaneously by a
technician while visually observing the pressure wave form
on an oscilloscope.

When the needle enters the artery, the solid plastic
casing surrounding the catheter is withdrawn, automatically
advancing the catheter up the artery to the subclavian.   No
fluoroscopic control is needed, since the catheter will not
pass beyond this point, due to the sharp angulation of the
artery and the rigidity of the catheter.   When this point is
reached, the pressure wave disappears and the catheter is
withdrawn two centimeters, where it remains for the rest of
the study.   The needle is withdrawn from the artery over the
catheter, and control measurements are performed.

A cardiac output determination may be made by injec-
ting dye into the antecubital vein and sampling through this
needle prior to introduction of the catheter.   However, in
many patients, since changes in cardiac output are of primary
interest, no absolute calibration against the dye method is
performed.   On completion of the control studies, the catheter
is removed from the strain gauge, filled with heparin, and

----

* SAFLEX , Romney Engineering & Manufacturing Company,
  Salt Lake City, Utah.
+ Sorenson Research Company, Salt Lake City, Utah

dead-ended. The catheter assembly is then taped to the fore-
arm and the patient is returned to his room. These catheters
have been left in place as long as 10 days, and in over 400
such procedures, most of which have been done by technicians,
no significant complications have resulted.

The next morning the patient goes to surgery, where
his catheter is once again connected to a pressure transducer
at a remote station in the operating room. Pressure
calibration is repeated by sampling the strain-gauge output
when it is exposed to 0 and 100 mm Hg pressure from a
mercury manometer through a saline flush system. From
that point on, the anesthesiologist can obtain a measurement
of pressure, stroke volume, heart rate, cardiac output, and
resistance by merely pressing an interrupt button on the
console at his side; the results are displayed back to him on
the oscilloscope of that console.

Other programs developed by Dr. William M. Stauffer,
in our laboratory, permit the anesthesiologist to enter other
pertinent information during the course of the procedure,
such as drugs administered and comments about the patient,
which become part of the computer-based record and can be
printed out at the end of the operation in the form of an integrated anesthesiology record on this patient.

After surgery, the patient is taken to a six-bed intensive care ward which contains a remote console, as shown in
Fig. 5.

At the top of this figure is shown a standard remote
computer input station with its memory oscilloscope, four-

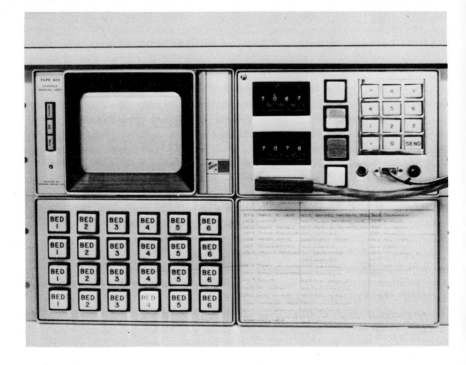

Fig. 5. Remote console located at nursing station in the intensive care ward.

digit switch, and 12-key decimal keyboard. This scope can be used both for computer writeout and for direct display of pressure or electrocardiographic wave forms from any bed. At the bottom is a second unit containing a bank of lights and a row of push-button switches used to indicate the bed from which wave forms are to be displayed. There are three lights

for each of the six beds. The green light indicates the computer is actively sampling data from that bed. The red and
yellow lights are used to alert the nurse that a change has
occurred in the patient occupying that bed.

To initiate a monitoring schedule on a patient, the
nurse or doctor presses the call button and then indicates the
bed number by pressing the corresponding number on the
decimal keyboard. The computer displays a list of options,
one of which is to initialize a schedule on the patient. When
the nurse presses the number corresponding to this option,
the computer will sample the next 64 heart beats on that
patient and determine the mean value and standard error
(S. E.) of the mean of each of the variables calculated from
the central aortic pressure pulse, as shown in Fig. 6.

```
     17.35
S . V .          52    5
H . R .          83    8
C . O .          44    6
S D U R         235   25
R S T            15    4
S Y  P          106    6
D I  P           66    4
V . P .          14
R . A .           2
R . R .          15
BED  NUMBER   5
  0  END, OR  BED  NO .
```

Fig. 6. Display of mean values and standard error of
the mean for stroke volume (S. V.), heart rate (H. R.), cardiac
output (C. O.), duration of systole (SDUR), resistance (RST),
systolic pressure (SYP), and diastolic pressure (DIP) measured
from central aortic pressure wave form on 64 heart cycles.
Mean venous pressure (V. P.), respiratory amplitude (R. A.),
and respiratory rate (R. R.) are derived from central venous
pressure signal.

In the first column are the mean values and in the
second column, the S. E. of the mean which then serves as a
basis for judging subsequent measurements on that patient.
If any subsequent measurement exceeds the expected mean
value for any variable by >3 S. E. , a red light turns on.

More subtle changes may be detected if they are systematic. If, for instance, stroke volume differs from its
expected mean value by 1 S. E. in the same direction on three
successive measurements, a trend is established and a yellow
light turns on. When a red or yellow light appears, the nurse
or doctor can press that light, which is also an interrupt
switch, and cause the computer to display an interpretation
of that light back on the memory oscilloscope, as shown in
Fig. 7.

In this case (Fig. 7), the variable furthest out of
tolerance is diastolic pressure. The last value, measured at
18:06, was 104 mm Hg, while the baseline value was 88 mm Hg.
To explain this rise in diastolic pressure, the nurse may choose
option 1, allowing her to enter clinical information which she
thinks might be pertinent to the physiologic observation. This
is entered by indicating whether it is a procedure, a condition,
or medication. Following this, an appropriate list under each
of these categories is presented and the nurse once again
chooses her specific entry from that list. This information is
then stored on disc as part of the patient's record for later
correlation with the physiologic information.

By pressing option 2, the nurse can review the course
of the patient over any arbitrary period of time. Under this

```
BED   3
DI  P

LAST        18. 6
  104
BASE        18. 2
  88
1   EXPLAIN
2   REVIEW
3   IGNORE
4   NEW BASE
5   WAVES
```

Fig. 7. Message displayed when the nurse presses red light to explain physiologic variation in a patient.

option the data are presented as shown in Fig. 8. The first column of numbers are the values for each of the variables measured at 17:37, and the second column are the values measured 2 min earlier. The user can page forward or backward, displaying values in this fashion to obtain information as to the time-course of events leading up to the physiologic change.

Any data that differ significantly from the baseline values are saved in the patient's file. The scheduling of measurements is done by the computer through an algorithm, which adjusts the interval between samples according to how stable the patient is. For example, if the patient is doing well, the interval between samples is made longer up to a maximum of 16 minutes, but if a change occurs in the patient's condition, that interval is shortened to 2 minutes on the next reading.

Another way in which the data may be reviewed by the nurse or doctor is to request a plot on the oscilloscope of the time-course of one or more variables over a time interval

```
        17.37    17.35
S.V.      53       52
H.R.      77       83
C.O.      42       44
SDUR     231      235
RST       16       15
SY  P    109      106
DI  P     65       66
V.P.      15       14
R.A.       1        2
R.R.      16       15
BED NUMBER 5
0 BAK,1 FOR,9 DEL
```

Fig. 8. Oscilloscope display under a review data option of program, showing two sets of readings 2 minutes apart for comparison.

requested by the user. Still another available aid for interpretation of physiologic change is provided through an option which permits the time-course of arterial pressure averaged over 16 heart beats at the time of the last measurement to be displayed on the oscilloscope and superimposed on the wave form recorded at the time of the baseline measurement. Changes in contour of these wave forms have provided useful information in detecting conditions, such as blood loss, at an early stage.

At the end of each 8-hour shift, a summary report is printed for each patient showing the mode values of each variable and the comments entered by the nurses. When a patient is discharged from the ward, his data are copied from disc to library tape and saved for subsequent analysis.

V. PATIENT SCREENING

An important part of the total system is a patient screening program. Every patient who is admitted to the

L. D. S. Hospital, with the exception of maternity and emergency patients, is screened using this program. When the
patient arrives at the hospital and registers in the admitting
office he is given a hospital record number. This number is
used by the computer system to generate a file of data for the
patient. Once the patient has received his registration forms
he is brought to an admitting laboratory where two samples
of blood and a urine sample are taken for analysis in the
chemistry laboratory. On leaving the admitting laboratory
the patient is brought to the computer screening laboratory.
A file is initiated on the patient by entering the patient's hospital number on the decimal keyboard at the terminal. A
nurse measures the patient's blood pressure, temperature,
respiration rate and enters these parameters along with age,
height, and weight in the patient's file.

Two on-line computer tests are then performed on the
patient. The first is a maximum breathing test where the
patient is required to take a deep breath and blow into a spirometer which measures both the total volume expired by the
patient (forced vital capacity), the volume expired after 1
second and two flow rates during the maximum expiration.
The analog signal generated by a potentiometer connected to
the spirometer is sent directly to the computer. Corrections
for temperature, barometric pressure, and calibration factors
are made by the computer and the results presented on the
display unit within 2 seconds after the test. Once the patient
has successfully performed this test, which usually requires
blowing into the spirometer at least twice in order to obtain
the best possible results, the patient is given a computerized

electrocardiogram (ECG) with the computer sampling the
output of the three vector signals from the ECG amplifier.
This test requires a series of eight electrocardiographic leads
to be connected to the patient. These leads are resolved by
the amplifier into an orthogonal lead system used for the
measuring of the electrical activity of the heart. The program
performs a pattern recognition on the data collected and
reports back to the screening technicians a classification of
an ECG pattern. This information is also stored in the
patient's file. Once the patient has completed his electrocardiogram he is taken to his room. Total time for these two
tests is approximately 5 minutes with the computer being used
for about 1 minute.

Other information entered into the patient's file includes
the results of the urine analysis and the hematology analysis,
and the blood chemistry tests run on a 12-channel autoanalyzer.
The 12-channel autoanalyzer is operated as an on-line terminal
which allows the computer to sample its output and store the
results directly into the patient's file. The urinalysis, as
well as the hematology results, are entered into the patient's
file through the keyboard at a remote terminal.

At the end of the day the technicians generate a report
from the patient's data by punching a card with the patient's
name and hospital number. The report generated for each
patient contains all the data which had been entered, either
automatically by the computer or keyed in from one of the
remote terminals. The program prints out the test results as
well as a problem list, that is, a listing of all values which

are outside normal limits. The reports are then distributed
to the nursing stations and placed on the patient's charts.
Subsequent data gathered on the patient during his stay in the
hospital are also recorded in the patient's file by the computer.
At time of discharge the file is taken from the active file,
which is stored on one of the magnetic discs, and transferred
to magnetic tape in the inactive file. At this time, or shortly
after, a discharge diagnosis is placed on the patient's record.
When the patient is readmitted to the hospital his record is
retrieved and pertinent information returned to the disc in the
active file.

VI. A TEACHING-TESTING PROGRAM FOR CORONARY-CARE NURSES

Any of the remote stations at the L. D. S. Hospital can
be used for teaching coronary-care nurses [4-7] using a
program developed for this purpose. The program simulates
the rhythm disturbances a patient with an acute episode of
ischemic heart disease might develop during his stay in a
coronary-care unit. It displays an electrocardiogram across
the face of the scope in the same way the nurse sees it on the
oscilloscopes of the intensive care unit, with the cathode ray
sweep inscribing the graph from left to right as the electrocardiogram is being generated by the computer. First, a
normal sinus rhythm is displayed when the program is called
from the remote station. On the second sweep, an abnormal
tracing is presented to the user. This tracing is randomly
selected by the computer from a transition matrix containing
15 arrhythmias. External noise can be simulated by the

computer and may appear at random in the tracings as 60-
cycle interference, muscle tremor, or, in some cases, even
suggesting a loose electrode. Below the tracing being displayed
a message on the scope offers the information that three possible courses of action can be taken: (1) a medication can be
given, (2) a procedure can be carried out, or (3) more
information about the patient's condition can be obtained
(Fig. 9). The nurse faces a series of problems as the case is
being presented to her – the first of these is to diagnose the
condition of the patient. If she cannot diagnose the rhythmn
being displayed, one of the above options allows her to call
for a consultation which causes the diagnosis to be displayed
in the form of a message on the scope above the tracing. Still
another option allows the student to ask for the optimal treatment and cause this to be displayed. She pays a price for

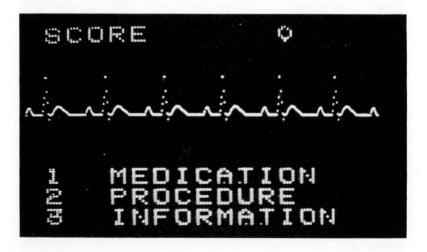

Fig. 9. Electrocardiogram and options for courses of
action.

this, however, since six points are subtracted from her score (see below) each time this option is used. In the same way, information regarding the patient's blood pressure can be obtained by selecting the proper option on the display.

Once a diagnosis is established, which may include rhythm, blood pressure, technical quality of the tracing, etc., action can be taken by choosing the medication or procedure option. If medication is indicated, the nurse may select a drug from a list offered to her by the program, which includes digitalis, vasopressors, atropine, isoproterenol, lidocaine, procainamide, and quinidine (Fig. 10). If a specific procedure is in order, such as cardioversion, carotid sinus pressure, or the use of a pacemaker, this can be entered through the numerical keyboard by pressing the numbered key corresponding to this option. If noise is present, it can be cleared by choosing the option labeled CHECK ELECTRODES. When a therapeutic decision is made and the corresponding action taken, a transition to a new condition will occur based on a random selection from the appropriate segment of the transition matrix, as explained below.

The program keeps a running score, based on the appropriateness of the decisions made, and continually displays this on the upper part of the scope (see below). If no decision regarding treatment is made by the nurse after two to four sweeps of the oscilloscope, the patient's condition will change again based on other elements in the transition matrix which reflect the expected natural course of the existing condition. If no treatment is instituted promptly in conditions such as ventricular fibrillation or hyperkalemia, a message on the

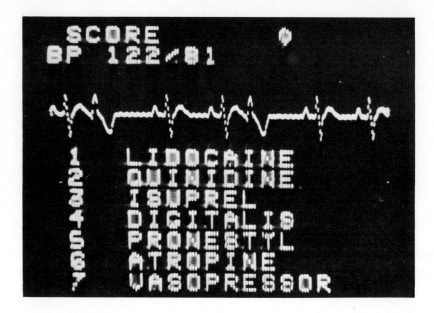

Fig. 10. Medication options. Score and blood pressure are also displayed.

scope will announce the patient's death after a short time. A new case can then be started or the session can be terminated.

At any point in the program the user can request a chart showing the course of events so far displayed, the blood pressure status at the time of each arrhythmia and whether the patient was taking digitalis (Fig. 11). The chart will also indicate the treatment given by the user and the best therapeutic approach to have taken under these circumstances (optimum decision, see below). This information is automatically displayed by the program after 10 consecutive changes in the patient's condition have taken place but can be requested by the student at any time. If, during the treatment, digitalis is given, the program must take this fact into account in sub-

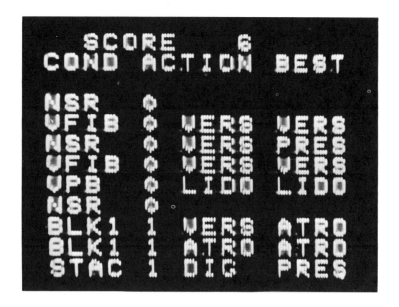

Fig. 11. Chart.

sequent therapeutic decisions since subsequent transitions
will be based on a different set of probabilities which reflect
the effect of digitalis. This feature will familiarize the user
with the effect of this drug on such conditions as the ventricular response to atrial fibrillation and the action of quinidine
sulfate and other drugs used in the treatment of arrhythmias.

For a patient receiving digitalis, the possibility often exists
that the arrhythmia is due to digitalis itself and requires
treatment which is quite different from that indicated in a
patient not receiving this drug.

The program is based on a tridimensional transition
matrix (Fig. 12). The condition of the patient at any given time
is represented on the Y axis and the treatment or lack of it
along the X axis. On the Z axis are the conditions in which

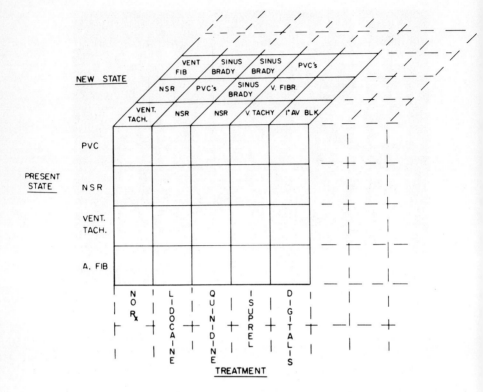

Fig. 12.   Transition matrix.

the patient with condition X is likely to find himself if he only
receives treatment Y.   A series of probability tables in the
program determine the conditions that may result from the
user's action.   For instance, if the patient has developed
arrhythmia A and the student chooses to institute therapy B,
there is a high probability that the patient will go to condition
D, a lower probability that he will go to condition E, a still
lower probability of F, and zero probability of going to any of
the other conditions in the table.   A random number is gener-

ated in the program to choose which condition according to these probabilities will be the new status of the patient.

To generate a random number, the computer samples the current reading of its internal 10-kc clock and masks out everything but the last six bits (this will be a number between zero and 77 octal). This number will be random because the time between clock readings is variable due to the fact that it includes the time for the student to make his decision. The algorithm by which the computer selects the next state involves comparing this random number to the first probability in the appropriate segments of the table. If this probability is less than the random number, the second probability from the table is added to the first and another comparison made. If the sum is greater than the random number, the state corresponding to the second probability is chosen. As a specific example, if condition A were atrial fibrillation with rapid ventricular response (which diminishes ventricular filling and causes a fall in cardiac output and systemic hypotension [8]) the best action would be to use the dc cardioverter. This is not the only available effective treatment, however, but the one that has the highest probability of restoring normal sinus rhythm and normal blood pressure under these circumstances. However, in spite of this being the optimal choice in most cases with this set of circumstances, the procedure may induce ventricular fibrillation, because of a nonsynchronized discharge in the vulnerable phase [9,10], or any other known or unknown factor [11]. Even if ventricular fibrillation does result, this treatment in general is the best choice and the student's score is increased accordingly. The same may apply to quinidine-induced ventricular fibrillation [12], procainamide-induced hypotension [13], or a junctional tachycardia secondary to digitalis therapy [14, 15]. In this teaching program all these factors are taken into consideration in the scoring mechanism and a positive number is added to the score when the decision made is a good one, regardless of what happens to the patient in the particular case. As another example to illustrate the point consider a hypotensive patient given isoproterenol when sinus bradycardia is present. In most cases the program will make him normotensive at the next transition. However, there is a real but small probability that ventricular tachycardia (or supraventricular with aberrant ventricular conduction) will result even though the score paradoxically increases. Similarly, a negative number is added to the score when the action taken is not a good one.

With each decision a new score (NS) is calculated from the old score (OS) according to the formula

$$NS = OS + 6(DX/DXM - 0.5) \qquad (1)$$

where DX is a decision function defined by

$$DX = PX - PRX \qquad (2)$$

PX (benefit factor) is the probability that the chosen treatment will result in transition to normal sinus rhythm and normal blood pressure, and PRX (risk factor) is the probability of the chosen treatment resulting in ventricular fibrillation or ventricular tachycardia (whichever is greater). DXM is the decision function for the optimal RX (the one having maximum DX).

In those cases in which no treatment is indicated, taking no action will increase the score. However, when an active decision is in order, it has to be made promptly since a delay in applying the appropriate measures may result in rapid deterioration of the patient's condition and finally his death (with an accompanying low score). This feature puts pressure on the student to make decisions quickly as he or she must do in the coronary-care ward. Thus, the program becomes a realistic simulation of the situations commonly seen in a coronary-care unit and allows the students to make decisions which affect the subsequent course of the simulation.

The probability tables currently used in this program are based on a review of the current literature on the subject and the author's experience. These tables are only approximations to the actual probabilities but they will be modified and improved as further pertinent data are collected from coronary-care wards; the transition matrix provides an explicit format for this data collection. The program is flexible enough that new drugs or procedures can be added to the matrix, others can be deleted or changed and new tracings can be generated to represent additional arrhythmias, when this is desirable.

Figure 13 shows a segment of a probability table corresponding to the specific situation of a patient with atrial flutter. In the first row, the symbol TAB12 references the computer to a location in magnetic core where this segment of the table is located, the 1 indicating that this table refers to a drug in the medication list and the 2 defining this drug as quinidine. If the student elects to administer quinidine to the patient,

```
PROBABILITY TABLE FOR QUINIDINE IN
ATRIAL FLUTTER

TAB12    OCT 40001013    NORMAL BP  - NO DIGITALIS
         OCT 20004013    LOW BP     - NO DIGITALIS
         OCT 6000        NORMAL BP  - DIGITALIS
         OCT 40001002    LOW BP     - DIGITALIS
```

Fig. 13. Probability table.

the program will reference one of the four cells in memory
that form this segment of the table, according to the patient's
condition at this time. The first and second and the fifth and
sixth octal digits in each row indicate the probability that the
administration of quinidine will cause the patient to go into the
state indicated by digits 3-4 and 7-8, respectively. For
instance, if this patient with atrial flutter receives quinidine
when his blood pressure is normal and he has already been
digitalized, the program will reference the third line of the
table segment shown. The octal digits 6000 indicate that there
is a 60/80 probability that he will go to condition 0 (normal
sinus rhythm) at the next transition and an implied 40/80 probability that his condition will not change. If he has not been
digitalized, the first line in this segment of the table will be
referenced and there will be 40/80 probability of reverting to
normal sinus rhythm (4000), a probability 10/80 of going to
condition 13, which is atrial fibrillation with rapid ventricular
response (1013), and an implied 30/80 probability that the
rhythm will not be affected unless further action is taken. The
second and fourth line in this segment illustrate the transitions
that may take place when the patient is hypotensive (condition
02 being atrial fibrillation with slow ventricular response).

Certainly a limiting factor in the quality of patient care in a coronary-care unit is the quality of the decisions made by the staff. This program is designed to give the nurse a concentrated experience in making these decisions based on realistic data. A program is only as good as its ability to represent reality both in terms of the variety of the arrhythmias presented, the probabilistic nature of the transitions made and the fact that these transitions are based on real observations. In any given clinical situation the therapeutic decision is based on the assumption that this case will behave like the average case in the same situation. In the simulation program, however, the user is made aware that there are other possible responses, as is often the case in real life, and is allowed to gain experience in making these vital decisions without risking someone's life until he has optimized his decision-making capabilities, as nearly as possible.

The practical use of this program in the training of nurses already working or being trained to work in coronary-care facilities during the past several months has been very satisfactory. More than 150 nurses trained and tested to date have shown definite improvement in their ability to make an adequate decision after properly evaluating the patient's situation in a short time, as evidenced by their ability to improve their scores using the simulation method.

In conclusion, it should be mentioned that as the simulation of the coronary-care unit becomes a more accurate reflection of reality it will also become a useful on-line tool for informing the nurse or the physician as to what action is the most adequate in a given situation. This will occur when machines become less expensive and the data base more adequate for performing this decision-making process.

VII. EFFECTS ON HOSPITAL PERSONNEL

It is interesting to reflect on the changes that have occurred in the attitudes and goals of the people involved in this project. Initially it was hoped that the computer monitoring, by relieving the nurse of some routine measurement duties, might provide her with some free time, and thus decrease the number of nurses required to care for these patients. However, this has not been the case. Even though the nurse is relieved from some of her monitoring and recording duties, she is busier than ever, as is the doctor. The reason for this lies in the fact that they now know much more about their patient, and are forced to make many more decisions than before when they were, to a greater extent, in the dark about what was going on physiologically.

Even though the physiologic data are screened to present only that information which indicates a statistically significant physiologic change, the job of interpreting this change and the intellectual task of deciding what to do about it is one we are not as yet qualified to perform well. Even with 2 years experience with this system, many situations still arise which not only the nurse but also the doctor have difficulty in interpreting. It is for this reason that we are accumulating, in parallel with the physiologic data, as much clinical information as possible, in the hope that in time we will develop sufficient correlative information to permit the computer to assist us in more accurate interpretation of the clinical meaning of the data with which we deal.

Although the monitoring system is continually evolving to include additional variables such as pH, pCO_2, and pO_2, which were recently added, even at this point in time it has proven its usefulness and does contribute to better patient care. Perhaps the best evidence of this is the fact that some surgeons doing open-heart surgery will now postpone a case if, for some reason, the computer monitoring system is not available.

This transition from emphasis on largely routine and somewhat mechanical activities to sometimes difficult intellectual effort is not an easy one for the nurse to make. It does require considerable retraining and shift of emphasis. The advent of the computer can be expected to bring equally drastic changes to the physician as well, as he begins to allocate more and more of the routine aspects of information storage, pattern recognition, and diagnosis to the machine, and finds himself spending more time dealing with creative and sometimes difficult new aspects of the world of medicine.

REFERENCES

1. H. R. Warner, "The Role of Computers in Medical Research," JAMA, 196, 944 (1966).

2. T. A. Pryor and H. R. Warner, "Time-Sharing in Biomedical Research," Datamation, 54 (April 1966).

3. R. M. Gardner and J. J. Ostlund, "Communication Systems for Remote Access to a Biomedical Digital Computer," Proc. 19th Ann. Conf. on Eng. in Med. & Biol., 1966, vol. 8, p. 141.

4. P. M. Yu, C. A. Imboden, Jr., S. M. Fox, III and
    T. Killip, III, "Coronary-Care Unit: A Specialized
    Intensive Care Unit for Acute Myocardial Infarction
    (Part II)," Mod. Conc. Cardiovasc. Dis., 34, No. 6
    (1965).

5. B. Lown, A. M. Fakhron, W. B. Hood, Jr., and
    G. W. Thorn, "The Coronary-Care Unit – New Perspec-
    tives and Directions," JAMA, 199, 188 (1967).

6. H. W. Day, "An Intensive Coronary-Care Area," Dis.
    of the Chest, 44, 423 (1963).

7. P. M. Yu, C. A. Imboden, Jr., S. M. Fox, III, and
    T. Killip, III, "Coronary-Care Unit: A Specialized
    Intensive Care Unit for Acute Myocardial Infarction
    (Part I)" Mod. Conc. of Cardiovasc. Dis., 34, No. 5
    (1965).

8. C. K. Friedberg, Diseases of the Heart, W. B. Saunders
    Co., Philadelphia, 1966, Vol. I, p. 536.

9. E. M. Ross, "Cardioversion Causing Ventricular
    Fibrillation," Arch. Int. Med., 114, 811 (1964).

10. H. T. Robinson and J. A. Wagner, "dc Cardioversion
    Causing Ventricular Fibrillation," Am. J. M. Sc., 249,
    300 (1965).

11. T. Killip, "Synchronized dc Precordial Shock for
    Arrhythmias," JAMA, 186, 1 (1963).

12. A. Selzer and H. W. Wray, "Quinidine Syncope –
    Paroxysmal Ventricular Fibrillation Occurring during
    Treatment of Chronic Cardiac Arrhythmias," Circ.,
    30, 17 (1964).

13. H. Schoolman, L. R. Pascale, L. M. Bernstein, and
    A. Littman, "Arterenol as an Adjunct to the Treatment
    of Paroxysmal Tachycardia," Am. Ht. J., 46, 146
    (1953).

14. A. Pick and A. Dominguez, "Non-Paroxysmal A-V
    Nodal Tachycardia," Circ., 16, 1022 (1957).

15. L. S. Dreifus, G. Bartolucci and W. Likoff, "Nodal
    Tachycardia – Etiology and Therapy," Circ., 22, 741
    (abstract) (1960).

11

Use of Automated Techniques in the Management of the Critically Ill *

Max H. Weil, Herbert Shubin, Lee D. Cady, Jr.,
Howard Carrington, Norman Palley, and Roy Martin

The Center for the Critically Ill and Shock Research Unit
University of Southern California and Hollywood
Presbyterian Hospital, Los Angeles, California

I. INTRODUCTION AND HISTORICAL PERSPECTIVE

Medical and surgical critical care facilities and post-anesthesia recovery units, which are now well established, have recently been complemented by additional intensive care units for management of trauma, respiratory insufficiency,

---

* Portions of this chapter are reprinted with permission of the publishers from the following articles: "Patient Monitoring and Intensive Care Units, " by M. H. Weil, H. Shubin, and D. Stewart, in Future Goals of Engineering in Biology and Medicine, edited by J. F. Dickson and J. H. U. Brown, (Academic Press, New York, 1969); Physical Arrangements at the Bedside in Support of Automated Systems for Patient Care, " by Howard Carrington, Herbert Shubin, Roy Martin, Norman Palley, and Max Harry Weil, published in IEEE Transactions on Biomedical Engineering, March, 1971; and, "Programming in the Medical Real-Time Environment, " by N. A. Palley, D. H. Erbeck and J. A. Trotter, published in AFIPS-Conference Proceedings, 37, 1970.

coronary episodes, and renal failure. Specialized medical, nursing, and technical personnel, competent monitoring devices, and a generous resource of supplies and equipment are pooled in such units to bolster both the efficiency and competence of medical care during periods of life-threatening illness.

The impact of this development and the wide use of intensive care facilities is vividly demonstrated by the current practice of the Los Angeles County General Hospital, in which 11 separate intensive care units provide 120 beds, approximately 5% of the total bed capacity of the hospital. In fact, this number is exclusive of additional beds provided in the postanesthesia recovery and coronary-care units. According to the Commission for Administrative Services in Hospital, between 3 and 5% of the total bed capacity in acute short-term hospitals is required for intensive or critical care [1].

The intensive care concept has evolved in the last 10 years as the first of five stages of progressive patient care [2, 3]. Its clinical function is to provide the most concentrated care, and thereby improve the survival of patients affected with life-threatening conditions. Many of the patients are admitted in coma and with shock. Specific disease states which underlie the medical and surgical catastrophes include pneumonia, drug overdose (commonly with suicidal intent), bleeding from an intestinal or stomach ulcer, diabetic coma, body burns, strokes, pulmonary and peripheral emboli, pulmonary edema, and serious disorders of the cardiac rhythm, particularly when they occur after a heart attack (myocardial infarction).

Development of intensive care facilities is in part a
direct outgrowth of the limited availability of highly specialized nursing personnel. There is a critical shortage of
professional nurses who are both well trained and devoted to
the general nursing care of seriously ill medical patients and
postoperative care of major surgical cases. Nursing talents
are pooled to assure maximal efficiency and expertise when
these are critical determinants of survival.

In the past 5 years there has been additional speciali-
zation of intensive care facilities in large medical centers.
Coronary care units, trauma units, renal dialysis units, and,
in Europe, "reanimation" or "resuscitation" units for treatment of drug overdosage, asphyxia, or poisoning, have come
into being. Patients are maintained in intensive care units
for an average of three days [4]. Although there is no quantitative documentation of apparent increases in survival,
there is little doubt that the availability of such units has been
life saving. The documented success of cardiac resuscitation
alone serves as a vivid example.

This chapter presents an overview of the problem of
designing automated systems for the care of critically ill
patients. The development of the USC Shock Research Unit
and the Center for the Critically Ill at the Hollywood Presbyterian Hospital are reviewed. Following a discussion of
physical facilities and monitoring devices, we discuss the
significant problems of computer programming for the real-
time environment of such a center.

A.   Physical Facilities

The intensive care unit is preferably located in close proximity to the operating suite, the central supply service, and the x-ray laboratory.   Ideally, 100 square feet are allowed for each bed, and a minimum of three and a maximum of eight beds are deemed optimal.   The space is air conditioned and generously supplied with routine and emergency sources of electric power.   The physical facility includes built-in monitoring devices, wall-mounted oxygen inlets, suction devices, and stands to facilitate intravenous administration of fluids.

B.   Personnel

In contrast to the average daily requirement of 5 hours of nursing service for general patient care (including the services of a vocational nurse, nurse's aide, and clerk), between 9 and 13 hours of such services are required for management of the critically ill.   In relation to less elaborately staffed general care facilities elsewhere in the hospital, the intensification of nursing coverage in the intensive care unit is regarded as mutually beneficial, since this protects the general care units from the crises of critical illnesses which impose unscheduled nursing loads.   The nurse specializing in intensive care must also be emotionally suited for work in an environment in which mortality is disproportionately high and major crises are daily occurrences.   These qualifications contrast with those of the private duty nurse, who formerly provided intensive care for the critically ill.   This "special" nurse functioned in a private practice relationship to patients.

By her very separation from routine responsibilities of general duty nursing in a well-organized hospital environment, the private duty nurse was actually deprived of special education and refined nursing experiences in respiratory care, cardiac resuscitation, monitoring techniques, and other technically refined methods which now represent basic skills of nurses serving in intensive care units.

Expert operation of the intensive care facility also requires the services of an array of paramedical specialists. One or more technologists and at least one part-time engineering (electronic) aide are usually needed. The medical supervision is provided by a physician who is skilled in general medicine and in clinical cardiopulmonary physiology. An anesthesiologist, a cardiologist, or a medically oriented surgeon typically leads the team. He is advised and assisted by part-time or consultant physicians representing the medical, surgical, and specialty services, including professional engineering personnel.

Technical personnel from ancillary services either train or assign staff, which functions in close relationship to the intensive care team. Included are technologists, who measure blood gases repetitively to guide the use of ventilators; laboratory technicians, who make other chemical or hematological measurements on blood, urine, and other biological fluids on a priority basis; radioisotope technicians, who measure blood volume; technicians, who obtain electrocardiograms and portable chest x-rays; and inhalation therapists, who service the respiratory equipment. In smaller units all

of these duties may be assigned to a competent technologist
who has had the advantage of multidisciplined training.

C. Limitations and Problems

Current problems facing the organization and operation
of intensive care units relate largely to the major commitment
of highly trained personnel and physical resources to the care
of a relatively small number of patients who require a
seemingly inexhaustible array of diagnostic and therapeutic
services.   The economic implications of this are partly
reflected in cost to patients.   In metropolitan Los Angeles the
charge for an intensive care bed in the four largest hospitals,
exclusive of the county hospital, ranges from $100-$200 per
day, not including the costs of laboratory services and medications.   General care costs in wards of comparable size
range from $50-$75 per day.   However, private duty nursing
on a 24-hour-a-day basis would actually result in costs approx-
imating those of the intensive care unit and yet not provide the
uniformly high level of professional supervision and ancillary
services provided in the intensive care units.

Space is a serious problem.   Personnel, supplies, and
large items of equipment are now crowded into an already
cramped area.   There are significant commitments of staff
for transcribing and tabulating information for the clinical
record and maintaining communication between service personnel, physicians, and patients' families.   A relatively large
number of employees must be housed in the unit for these
purposes, and the intensive care unit is therefore congested.
Major advances in systematized, integrated operation using

automated procedures which would obviate the need of some
personnel are greatly needed [5, 6].

Staffing for intensive care units is not usually a problem, since nurses are particularly attracted to intensive
care duty. Yet this creates a debit of staff availability for
other units of the hospital and adds to the more general problem of hospital staffing. A major consideration is the cost
of training and retraining as rapid technological advances are
made. In our own unit at the Hollywood Presbyterian Hospital
a minimum of 6 work weeks and half of the time of the super-
visor are required before the nurse or technologist can function independently. Since the average duration of employment
in our hospital is less than 1-1/2 years, more than 12% of the
total effort is expended on a continuing basis for preliminary
and in-service training, exclusive of additional investments
in the training of personnel for centers which are being established in other hospitals. There has not yet been enough
time for the wider development of formal training programs
and facilities for nurses or technicians.

Efficiency of operation is needed to reduce the workload of technicians and nurses. Present manual methods of
data keeping and the time required for manual monitoring
impose ever-increasing demands on staff, particularly
during the night hours and weekends, when staffing is minimal.

D. Monitoring

Electrocardiographic amplifiers and oscilloscopes are
routinely used for continuous display of the electrocardiogram.
The arterial pulse rate, blood pressure, and respiratory rate

are monitored on a routine basis, preferably at intervals of
15 minutes. Rectal or esophageal temperature is also routinely
monitored. A detailed record of the intake and output of fluids
is maintained. Bedside laboratory studies include measurements of specific gravity of urine, urine sugar or acetone in
diabetic patients, and occult blood in the gastric aspirate or
stool. Specific inventories of nonnumerical observations of a
patient's condition are recorded, such as state of alertness,
skin color, evidence of pain, quality of the arterial pulse, and
the alterations in depth of respiration. In a minority of center
the electroencephalogram is monitored, particularly in the
case of patients who are in coma. Body weight may be measured at intervals of 8 hours or less, using frame-mounted or
floor-recessed scales or load cells.

E.   Instrumentation for Emergency Treatment

Inhalation and resuscitation equipment is maintained in
constant readiness at the bedside. For correction of serious
defects in the rhythm of the heart, cardiac defibrillators and
pacemakers are immediately available. Cardiac massage,
previously performed by manual methods and without machi-
nery, is now partially or even totally mechanized by use of
hand-operated or electrically driven precordial compressors.
Suction devices are used for care of tracheostomy sites, chest
tubes, and gastrointestinal aspiration. Patients in whom
generalized nervous depression (coma) or a defect in nerve or
muscle function accounts for paralysis of respiratory muscles
or patients who have advanced cardiac or pulmonary disabili-
ties may be unable to maintain adequate oxygen and carbon

dioxide exchange. Under these circumstances artificial ventilation must be maintained. The lungs are inflated and deflated
with warmed and humidified mixtures of oxygen and air at
established cycling rates. Intermittent positive pressure
ventilators, initially introduced for bronchodilator treatment
of asthmatic conditions, have been adapted for this use. More
recently, volume-controlled ventilators such as the Swedish
Engstrom respirator have been preferred, since optimal
volumes of gas are not as reliably delivered by the pressure-
regulated devices. Specialized catheters, adapters, and
mechanical flushing devices are used to maintain patency of
venous or arterial catheters or arterial-venous shunts. Motor-
driven pumps are used for infusion of medications or fluids.

Other specialized devices developed in our own center
are discussed in Section II.

F. Current Status of Automation

Since the manual operation of an ever-increasing number of devices and the expanding chores of record keeping
have further infringed on the nurses' already greatly limited
time for direct patient care, a new measure of efficiency is
direly needed to facilitate both patient monitoring and routine
management. With but a few salient exceptions, automated
techniques are not widely used at present. Rectal and esophageal thermistors are commonly employed for temperature
measurement in patients, particularly when hypothermia is
used in conjunction with cardiac surgery or neurosurgery.
Blood pressure is sometimes measured by use of automated

analog devices employing automatic cuff inflators and indirect
auscultatory techniques [7, 8], but this technique has limited
reliability, particularly during shock, when the peripheral
pulse is very feeble. Measurement of intra-arterial pressure
by an external transducer, such as a strain-gauge manometer,
or by a needle or catheter-tip transducer is much more accurate, but is not generally used because of the potential injury
attendant on the insertion of catheters directly into arteries.
Central venous pressure is usually measured with a water
manometer, but it may also be measured with a strain-gauge
transducer [9]. Densitometers are now widely used in
research centers for measurement of cardiac output by dye
dilution techniques. Such instruments are sometimes operated
in conjunction with special-purpose analog computers, which
greatly facilitate computation of cardiac output, circulation
time, and central blood volume [10]. Estimates of cardiac
output have also been obtained by calculation of stroke volume
from components of the arterial pressure wave, but these
have not been fully validated for use under pathological conditions [11]. The Fick principle, based on measurement of
oxygen consumption, and spectrophotometric determination of
blood oxygen in both the pulmonary and the peripheral arteries
have been used by Guyton et al. [12], for assessment of
cardiac output, but this requires even more extensive catheterization procedures. Commercially available automated
chemistry devices have been used for rapid chemical determinations on blood, including sugar, sodium, potassium,
creatinine, and lactic acid. Indeed, mobile units are available
for electrochemical measurements of pH, pCO_2, and pO_2.

Even measurement of pO_2 without withdrawal of blood samples has recently become feasible with the introduction of catheter-mounted microelectrodes, but these have not been perfected for clinical use.

Clinicians are concerned not only with acquisition, but also with the practical analysis of the data which are obtained in order to assure their immediate usefulness at the bedside. Although the experience with "on-line" operations is extremely limited, comparable data have been efficiently managed "off line" by automated methods in a research environment [13-15]. An automatic transducer system and digital computer for simultaneous measurement of blood pressure, pulse, respiration, and temperature during anesthesia have been described by Wilber and Derrick [16]. In our laboratory a combination of automated sensors and amplifiers with output transmitted to a central processor has extended the usefulness of on-line measurements [17].

G. The University of Southern California Shock Research Unit

The development of a system which provides a relatively comprehensive inventory of the patient's physiological condition using a combination of automated sensors and a digital computer has been described elsewhere [18, 19]. In brief review, efforts by our group began a number of years ago, when plans were made for the intensive study and care of patients in shock in a specialized research unit at the Los Angeles County General Hospital. In November 1961 a four-bed shock research unit was opened at this hospital under

the auspices of the University of Southern California Medical
School and supported by the John A. Hartford Foundation of
New York. In mid-1963 a digital computer serving as part of
a data acquisition system was installed. This system consis-
ted of an IBM 1710 process control computer equipped with an
analog-to-digital converter, interval timer, 2-million-charac-
ter disc file, card read punch, manual entry units, plotter,
and output typewriter. The next 2 years were devoted to the
development of an automated data acquisition and display
system to serve the clinical needs of this ward as well as the
need for efficient accumulation of data for purposes of clinical
research.

In 1967 the unit was transferred to the Hollywood
Presbyterian Hospital, where it was integrated with a new,
modern intensive and coronary care unit, the Center for the
Critically Ill. The IBM 1710 computer was replaced with an XDS
Sigma 5 and a number of new instruments were developed and in-
stalled, as described in Section II.

II. PHYSICAL ARRANGEMENTS AT THE BEDSIDE IN
SUPPORT OF AUTOMATED SYSTEMS FOR PATIENT CARE

A. Introduction

The Center for the Critically Ill is a joint development
of the Shock Research Unit of the University of Southern California School of Medicine and the Hollywood Presbyterian
Hospital. This center is a forerunner of a much needed
interdisciplinary effort which provides a team of not only
physicians, nurses, and medical technologists, but biochemists,
mathematicians, engineers, electronic technicians, program-

mers, and statisticians, all of whom are concerned with the delivery of more competent and efficient care to critically ill patients.

The shock ward provides a facility for comprehensive monitoring and treatment of very ill patients, using automated techniques. Operation of monitor and servo controlled effector modules is centered in a medium-size digital computer system (XDS Sigma 5).

In addition to the shock ward, the Center for the Critically Ill includes a six-bed coronary-care unit, a nine-bed intensive care unit, and a 23-bed concentrated care unit. This latter unit provides a buffer for the other higher level care units, thus insuring their optimal availability and use. The purpose of the next section is to describe the operational considerations that guided our group in the design of the two-bed shock ward. One of the two symmetrical bed units is shown in Fig. 1.

B.   Physical Design of the Unit

An engineer rarely has the opportunity to design a special service center in a hospital from its very beginning. Many of the parameters, such as room boundaries, number of beds, spacing between beds, and space for special services and equipment, are previously specified. Most often, the designer must modify existing spaces within fixed and often undesirable boundaries. The Shock Research Unit, when developed as a component of the Center for the Critically Ill, required such a compromise. The room, which is 15 by 34 feet, has space cutouts for dumbwaiters, vertical pipe chases,

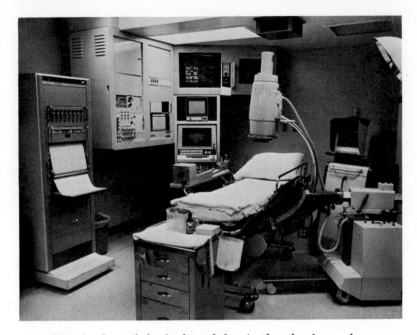

Fig. 1. One of the bed modules in the shock ward.

bed pan cleaners, and other utilities. The narrow width
precluded any options with respect to placement of the two
beds and required their long axis to be aligned with the long
axis of the room.

An accoustical ceiling, which lies below the ventilation
ducting and 8 feet 6 inches above the floor, contains recessed
fluorescent light fixtures. Dimmer controls allow a full range
of light intensity from 10 to 100 foot candles. Wall outlets for
oxygen, compressed air, suction and electric power, are
provided in the end walls for ready availability at the head of
each of the two beds.

C. Installation of the Two Beds

The design of the beds and the manner in which they
are positioned (Fig. 1) represent a compromise to secure
patient comfort, accommodate bedside personnel, provide
space for major items of equipment, and still fit into the space
available. The beds, which were designed collaboratively with
the Stryker Corporation, * are 30 inches wide. Though they
limit movement by the patient, they allow full access to the
patient from either side. The height of the bed usually is
30 inches, but adjustment by which the bed is elevated or
lowered 4 inches is provided to accommodate comfortably the
variable height of the bedside personnel. The head and the
foot of the bed may be separately elevated, the bed may be
separately elevated or lowered, and the bed may be tilted,
raising either the head or the foot.

The precarious condition of patients treated in this
ward is such that even their transfer from one bed to another
imposes a major, and even life-threatening hazard. The
patient is therefore kept on one multipurpose bed until his
condition is stabilized. To guide the placement of catheters
in central veins and arteries, and in the heart itself, a portable fluoroscopic image intensifier is routinely used. We

---

* Provided through the courtesy of the Stryker Corporation of
Kalamazoo, Michigan.

employ a Siemens Siremobil. * A "C" arm and the large base
of the image intensifier unit must be accommodated by the bed.
To permit passage of the x-ray beams, a radiolucent mattress
made of 3-inch-thick polyurethane foam is used. Together
with its waterproof cover, the mattress is very uniform in its
nominal absorption of radiation. The surface is movable on
longitudinal tracks, permitting the patient's body to be positioned for optimal viewing in the field of the image intensifier.

D. Side-Arm Instrument Supports

The instrumentation for immediate bedside use is
supported on a stainless steel structure (Fig. 2). Support
tubing is cantilevered from the floor at the head end of the bed
space. These tubes, which serve as supports for both sides
of the bed, swing laterally away from the bed. They also may
be extended along each side of the bed or telescoped together
using pairs of linear bearings. This design facilitates posi-
tioning of a 30-inch stainless steel and lucite tray in close
proximity to any desired body location.

All wires are led from the bedside by way of an open
gutter along the fixed section of the horizontal tubes to the
instrumentation island. Also along the gutter and facing the
floor is a conventional three-wire plug mold providing power
and ground at 6-inch intervals.

The side arms support pressure transducers, densitometers for dye dilution measurements, pumps for infusion

------

* Manufactured by Siemens Aktiengesellschaft.

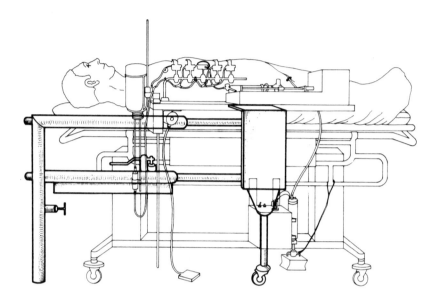

Fig. 2. Bedside structure for support of transducers, pumps, urinometer, and other instrumentation.

and/or withdrawal of blood, fluids, medication, a flush system for vascular catheters, and urinometers. The urinometer consists of a cylinder into which urine is delivered by a catheter which is routinely inserted into the patient's bladder. Urine volume is sensed in terms of the hydrostatic pressure of the fluid column in the cylinder acting through an air isolation section on a pressure transducer (Fig. 3). The computer tallies the volumes, periodically "dumps" the collected urine into another receptacle, and displays the volume of urine flow over both the preceding 5 and 60 minutes, on a constantly updated basis. An earlier model of the urinometer was described by Meagher [21].

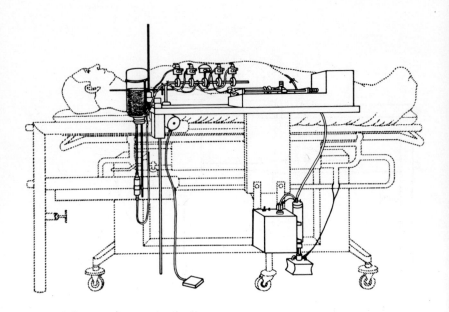

Fig. 3. Urinometer which utilizes a computer system
for automatic measurement of urine flow.

Automated blood infusion-withdrawal units for use at
the patient's bedside have been developed (Fig. 4). Samples
of blood are withdrawn from one of three catheters (right
atrium, pulmonary artery, aorta), or fluids are infused into
the atrial catheter. A flush system, under computer control,
is provided to keep catheters patent. Air operated valves
manufactured by BIO-LOGICS[*] at sites near the patient's body
are used in conjunction with more remote solenoid valves.
This arrangement obviates serious problems of electrical
safety. No stopcocks or loosely supported sections of plastic

---

[*] Salt Lake City, Utah.

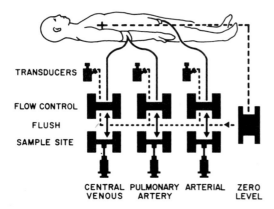

TRANSDUCERS

FLOW CONTROL

FLUSH

SAMPLE SITE

CENTRAL   PULMONARY   ARTERIAL   ZERO
VENOUS   ARTERY   LEVEL

Fig. 4. Automatic system for controlling withdrawal of
blood and infusion of fluid. This device also provides connection to automated devices for measuring blood gases (pH,
PCO_2, PO_2), blood volume, and chemical measurements in
blood.

tubing are used in the new units which are attached to the bedside support structure.

E. Transducer-Flush System

The three intravascular catheters routinely used by us
are connected to Statham P23, Dd, Db, or Gb transducers,
which are attached with plastic and stainless steel clamps to
the bedside support structure. Care is taken to assure minimal dead space between catheter and transducer in the interest
of optimal frequency response. A pressure of 290 mm Hg is
maintained on the surface of a saline reservoir. This provides
the pressure head for intermittent flushing of the catheters.
The saline enters into the catheter at a point distal to the
strain-gauge transducer so as to preclude errors due to ther-
mal shift.

Because of the special hazard of air embolization, a microswitch is used to sound an alarm when more than 80% of the saline has been removed from the reservoir. A check valve also precludes a flow of air from the reservoir to the catheters when volume in the reservoir is depleted. A foot-switch operated solenoid pinch valve on the flush line serves as another safety device so that fluid is delivered only on positive command. For calibration, a pressure of 200 mm Hg is automatically delivered to the saline surface in the flush bottle and, in turn, to the transducers. This provides a very convenient reference pressure for the self-balancing amplifiers which were developed by our group, and previously described by Martin [23].

F. Instrument Island

The head of each bed is placed 48 inches from the end wall to permit access to the patient from all four sides. An instrument "island" which is the same width and height as the bed, and 6 inches in depth, adjoins the head of the bed (Fig. 5). The island is formed by two metal boxes stacked on top of one another and the unit is encased with formica on plywood, except for the side facing the end wall. The lower (electrical) and upper (plumbing) boxes are readily entered by removing metal covers on the face toward the end wall. All connections to amplifiers or preprocessors are made through connectors on the sides of the island. Pressure lines for the air-operated valves emerge from the sides of the upper box, which also contains fixtures and plumbing for oxygen, air, and suction.

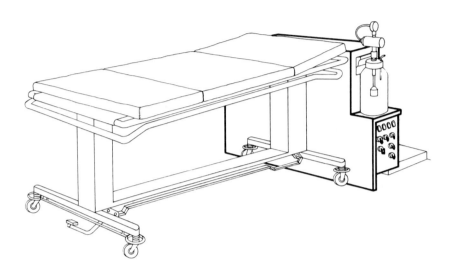

Fig. 5. Instrument island which provides site for utilities, electrical and pressure connections, and support for
the head of the bed while preserving access to the head of
the bed for patient resuscitation.

Connecting the instrument island to the wall is a flat

multichannel metal duct which provides ideal separation and

efficient protection of all the instrumentation lines. This duct

is covered by a 1/4-inch metal plate which permits ward staff

access in this area. Conduit connects each of the two islands

to the instrument control rack, and on through the ceiling to

the computer which is located in an area immediately above

the shock ward.

G. Instrument, Rack, Display, and I/O Devices

At present, the manual operation of the bedside devices,

amplifiers, and preprocessors precludes remote location of

major devices. As electrical-mechanical interfaces are
perfected, this will undoubtedly be facilitated. A large rack
and control panel is located 36 inches from the side of the bed
and adjacent to the recorder shown in Fig. 5, thus permitting
personnel to remain at the side of the patient, even when they
momentarily turn away from him to adjust the controls by
which the system is operated. A display module contains a
digital patient-status display scope, a four-channel raw-data
signal display, an XDS 7555 keyboard/CRT unit, and a
Tektronix 611 storage scope. The typewriter component of
the 7555 terminal is maintained at 36 inches for optimal use by
the operator as he is standing in front of it. The racks and
display modules extend from a level of 40 inches above the
floor to the ceiling. The space underneath these installations
is reserved for mobile equipment. The components of the
instrument rack and especially the amplifiers and recorders
are of modular construction and are readily replaced by plug-
in units. The equipment is operationally tested every 24 hours
to insure instant readiness.

III. PROGRAMMING IN THE MEDICAL REAL-TIME ENVIRONMENT

A. Introduction

The adoption of the general purpose digital computer
as an accepted tool in clinical medical practice has lagged far
behind the predictions of several years ago. Hospital information systems, including off-line analysis of patient data,
still constitute the major applications of computers in clinical

facilities [25]. Most patient monitoring in the recently
developed specialized coronary-care and intensive care units
is performed by special-purpose analog devices.

As in many other computer applications areas, there
is an ample selection of available digital hardware adequate
to the patient monitoring task. Interface hardware including
transducers, preprocessors, automated chemical analyzers,
and display devices of the required capability and reliability
are now becoming available. The software interface remains
the major barrier to clinical acceptance of the digital computer. It is not the programmer who will utilize a patient monitoring system, but the physician, nurse, and laboratory
technician. They may not appreciate the computer system
complexity nor forgive its idiosyncracies [26].

A major effort at the Shock Research Unit has been to
make the computer system transparent to the clinical staff
and the medically trained occasional programmer. In all
interactions between the clinical staff and the computer system
elaborate and unnatural coding schemes are avoided. All
instructions, lists, and alternatives are displayed by the
computer at the bedside with computer jargon replaced by
medical jargon. Often, computer system efficiency must be
traded for this improvement in the physician's or nurse's
understanding and acceptance of a procedure.

B.   General System Description

The primary monitoring functions are accomplished
by analog transducers attached to the patient which directly

sense physiological activity [27]. The resultant electrical signals, such as ECG and arterial and venous pressure wave forms are amplified and displayed at the bedside on a multi-channel oscilloscope, shown at D in Fig. 6. Analog signal conditioners perform some preprocessing, including the derivation of the heart rate and detection of the R wave from the ECG signal, and of respiration rate from the venous pressure signal. The outputs of these conditioners and amplifiers are passed to a multiplexer and A/D converter. In some cases, as in the reading of temperatures, a single-point analog read suffices and the digital processing consists in multiplying the converted voltage by the proper factor. The derivation of other parameters such as systolic and diastolic pressures and arterial dp/dt involves more complex digital procedures. The output of laboratory test devices, now in various stages of automation, for the monitoring of blood chemistry values, such as pO_2, pCO_2, and pH, are also input as analog signals. Another category of monitoring functions includes cardiac output [28] and blood volume determinations, the latter being calculated from the dilution of radioactive tracers in successive patient blood samples. The primary signals and the routinely displayed derived variables are shown in Table I.

Automatic monitoring programs are run at a frequency which is a property of the particular program and varies from once a minute for heart rate to once in 15 minutes for temperatures. Other programs, such as those involved in the determination of cardiac output, are called up by use of the keyboard as needed.

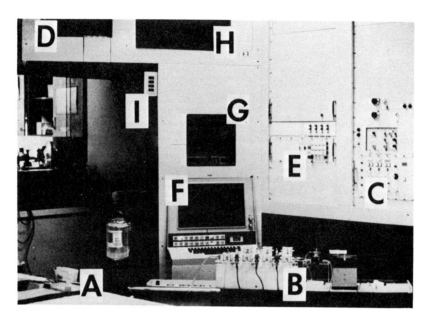

Fig. 6. Bedside displays and instrumentation. (A) bed
and instrument island; (B) transducers and interface; (C)
transducer amplifiers; (D) analog display; (E) analog display
controls; (F) keyboard/CRT terminal; (G) graphic display;
(H) status display; (I) alarm lights.

While the monitoring, analysis, and display of current
patient parameters is in itself an important task, if this were
the only function the system were called on to perform, a
sufficient number of special-purpose analog devices would
serve as well. However, the ability to store the monitored
data in highly structured form and to retrieve, manipulate,
and display the stored data in a variety of modes and post
facto rearrangements provides one of the justifications for
the use of a digital system.

TABLE I

Displayed Variables in Relation to Primary Signals

	Primary signal	Sensor	Displayed variable
1	Electrocardiogram	Electrode	a. heart rate b. maximum and minimum beat-to-beat interval c. standard deviation of beat-to-beat interval
2	Arterial or left ventricular pressure	Strain gauge transducer	a. systolic pressure b. diastolic pressure c. mean pressure (arterial) d. variation between highest and lowest systolic pressures in read interval e. pulse rate f. pulse deficit g. dp/dt of ventricular pressure pulse h. interval from onset of electrical to onset of mechanical systole
3	Venous pressure, central	Strain gauge transducer	a. mean pressure b. respiratory rate
4	Pulmonary artery pressure	Strain gauge transducer	a. systolic pressure b. diastolic pressure c. mean pressure
5	Temperature	Thermistor	a. rectal b. skin right toe c. skin left toe d. ambient air
6	Urine output	Strain gauge transducer	a. urine output last 5 min. b. urine output last hour c. cumulative volume

7	Optical density of blood	Densitometer	a. cardiac output b. cardiac index c. work done by heart d. stroke work e. vascular resistance f. central blood volume g. mean circulation time h. appearance time
8	Radioactivity of blood samples	Scintillation counter	a. plasma volume b. red cell volume
9	Manual input of raw data and calibration factors	Video terminal	a. PO_2 b. PCO_2 c. pH, H^+ concentration d. bicarbonate e. oxygen saturation f. lactate
1, 2, 3, 5	as above		alarm signals
2, 3, 7, 8, 9	as above		probability of survival

An elaborate alarm system is under development
which makes extensive use of the patient data file. The system
employs multivariate statistical techniques to examine the
simultaneous values of seven physiological variables and
compares them to equivalent sets monitored 5, 15, 30, and 60
minutes previously. Estimates are calculated on the probability of occurrence of these sets of values and changes, and
the system reports unusual changes to the ward staff. In
addition, critical processes such as the infusion of fluids and
medications may be automatically halted.

The patient monitoring system as implemented uses
an XDS Sigma 5 computer with a core memory size of 24K,
32 bit words. This system utilizes standard XDS peripherals
including digital I/O, A/D converter, D/A converter, a
3-million-byte disc drive, two seven-track tape drives, line
printer, card reader, and five keyboard displays (Fig. 7).

Data is obtained from the analog and digital inputs,
and from the keyboard displays. Once collected, processed,
and stored in a patient's file on the disc, it is retrieved and
stored or displayed on a variety of devices serving distinct
purposes. Depending on the device, this is done either automatically (scheduled) or on request. Most communication
between the medical staff and the machine is conducted through
the keyboard display (shown at F in Fig. 6). From these
devices the ward staff can start monitoring procedures, store
textual data, call for computation and analysis of the patient
data, and retrieve information from old patient files. A
special function key loads a program to display a list of other

A VARIETY OF DEVICES PERMITS DEVELOPMENT OF OPTIMAL DISPLAY AND CONTROL TECHNIQUES

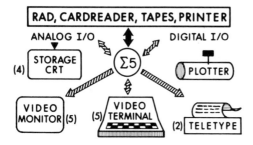

Fig. 7. Computer hardware configuration.

most commonly used programs (Fig. 8). The user then responds with his choice. The program selected may display data from a file, or present the user with another list representing a lower level of choices. Selections from these lists are indicated by entering the item number. The physiological status of each patient is displayed above his bed on a large-screen TV monitor (H in Fig. 6) driven by a character generator. A close-up of this display is shown in Fig. 9. This display includes the current values of 25 of the most important monitored variables.

The patient monitoring software is a library of applications programs, written in FORTRAN, functioning within a comprehensive executive system. Among the services provided to the applications programs by the executive are facilities for dynamic scheduling and loading of program modules. Other services include a data management system, and a variety of interfaces to I/O devices.

```
                    MENU

        ENTER BED NUMBER

        ENTER PROGRAM NUMBER

           1)  HEMODYNAMIC DATA SUMMARY
           2)  CARDIAC OUTPUT LIST
           3)  TEMPERATURE DATA SUMMARY
           4)  URINE OUTPUT SUMMARY
           5)  BROWSING PROGRAM

           6)  WARD STATUS REPORT
           7)  PATIENT ADMISSION
           8)  HISTORY
           9)  PHYSICAL EXAMINATION
          10)  LIST OF NURSES' NOTES

          11)  LIST OF LABORATORY STUDIES
          12)  PATIENT DISCHARGE
          13)  PROGNOSTIC INDEX
          14)  PATIENT FILE PRINTOUT
          15)  TREND PLOT

          16)  PATIENT FILE RETRIEVAL
```

Fig. 8. Displayed list of most commonly used programs.

The executive software is built on standard packages provided by XDS with some subtle but important differences. The operating system package chosen, while allowing for a real-time task, did not specifically allow for any sophisticated form of multiprogramming. This was available at a significant cost in core and disc memory space, but still was not adequate. The description and use of the necessary extensions made to the operating system are the subject of this section.

```
19/0517   STATUS        BED 1        BED 2

SYS/DIA                 64/37        96/58
MAP                     45           72
VEN                     6            8
HR/PDEF                 84/ 3        98/ 0
RESP                    17           22

RECT/AMB                34.6/25.4    37.1/25.4
TOE L/R                 24.8/24.3    24.9/25.3
UR5/UR60                   6/39         0/28

DAY/TIME                19/0201      19/0317
CI                      1.9          1.8
AT/MCT                  14/28        11/25
RESIST                  1347         2227

HCT/TIME                29/0210      19/0329
PH/PCO2                 7.31/51      7.49/24
PO2/SAT                   71/96      278/100

PV/TIME                 58/0224      29/0346
RCM/TIME                22/0224      19/0346
LAC/TIME                3.4/0217     2.9/0338
```

Fig. 9. Close-up of status display showing 25 of the derived measurements. The time is shown for measures which are made on demand, such as cardiac index (CI).

C.   Extended System Functions

Communication between FORTRAN application programs and the extended system functions is provided by a set of system interface routines (Table II). They are written in assembly language, and accessed through FORTRAN subroutine calling sequences in the applications programs. These functions provide the following facilities.

TABLE II

System Interface Routines

Subroutine name and function	Parameters
ANA Analog input	1. Interval between samples (in 1/500 of a second) 2. Number of samples 3. Present sample index 4. Wait/return code and buffer size 5. Number of channels 6. Array of channel numbers 7. Input data buffer 8. Return priority
ANAOUT Analog output	1. Output control 2. Channel number 3. Voltage
AQUIT Analog input halt	
CCIWR Status display write	1. Format statement number 2. , . . . , n) list of output variables
DELAY Precision delays	1. Time delay in 1/500 of a second
DELETE Delete scheduled program	1. Bed number 2. Name of program to be deleted 3. Error return
DIGIN Digital input	1. File or bed number 2. Array of words corresponding to digital input lines
DIGOUT Digital output	1. File or bed number 2. Line number 3. on/off code

Subroutine name and function	Parameters
GETDAT Patient file data retrieval	1. File or bed number 2. Summary name 3. Time desired or position code 4. Number of values requested 5. Names of the values 6. Array for data 7. Indicator for textual information 8. Error return 9. Intercall location pointer
IWAIT Wait for external interrupt	1. Number of interrupt to be armed 2. Return priority
KDRD Keyboard/display read	1. Format statement number 2. Parameter being read
KDWR Keyboard/display write	1. Format statement number 2. , . . . , n) list of output variables
PINIT Start program	1. File or bed number 2. Name of program to be started 3. Time between executions 4. Multipurpose variable passed to program
PRIOR Set program priority	1. Desired priority
PUTDAT Store patient data	1. File or bed number 2. Summary name 3. Time to be stored with data 4. Number of values being stored 5. Names of the values 6. Values to be stored 7. Indicator for textual summaries 8. Error return
TIME Get or set time	1. Get/set indicator 2. Time of day
TTWR Write on ward teletype	1. File or bed number 2. Format statement number 3. , . . . , n) list of output variables

(1) <u>Scheduling of program initiation frequency and
sequencing</u>. The system must be capable of initiating many tasks such as data analysis and control
programs without operator intervention. In addition, this capability is desirable in that it removes
sequencing and program initiation from application
programs.

(2) <u>Scheduling and interleaving of real-time data I/O</u>.
One of the major problems of real-time medical
applications is long-duration low-frequency analog
inputs. These frequencies and durations vary
from signal to signal. A scheduling structure is
required to facilitate concurrent analog data input
for many analysis programs and processing of that
data.

(3) <u>Dynamic system and user control of execution
priority</u>. A variety of tasks must be concurrently
served by the same processor. These tasks vary
widely in complexity and rate of execution, depen-
dence on I/O, and relation to the welfare of the
patient. A desirable feature is to allow the priority
of execution of these tasks to be dynamically altered
as a function of the type of processing, and as a
function of the patient condition as determined by
analysis programs or clinical staff.

(4) <u>Queuing of executing programs at priority levels</u>.
If dynamic priority reassignment is to be allowed
with a limited number of priorities, then it is

necessary to provide the capability for queuing
multiple programs at each priority level to insure
that executions can run to completion.

(5) Dynamic relocation of program at load time.
Since the system must be capable of loading program modules quickly and provide an efficient use
of core memory, it is necessary that the object
code for each task be stored in a form with all
references satisfied, yet with the capability of
being loaded dynamically through a relocating
loader.

(6) Data management. Patient management in the
critical care environment requires on-line sequential and random access to the entire patient file.
The components, and the organization of these
files, vary with changes in monitoring requirements. Consequently, a method must be provided
to associate a unique description with each file.

D. Applications Programs

The following description of the hemodynamic monitoring programs, FUZ1 and HEMO, will be used to illustrate
some of the unique capabilities afforded the FORTRAN application program by the system. HEMO reads arterial, venous,
and pulmonary arterial pressure wave-form data, and the
outputs of the electrocardiogram (ECG) preprocessor. From
these primary signals, 15 measures are derived and stored
in the patient file. Other programs retrieve and display this

information automatically and on demand. This monitoring
program normally runs once each 5 minutes (normal mode)
but optionally may be run once each minute (acute mode) or be
surpressed entirely (wait mode) under bedside control.

The hemodynamic program is quite large, and any
combination of primary signals may not be available at the
scheduled initiation of the program. Thus, in order to avoid
loading the program unnecessarily, it is not started directly
by the program scheduler (PSKED). Instead, a small trigger
program, FUZ1, the listing of which is shown in Fig. 10 is
scheduled to run once each minute. Applications programs as
started by PSKED are not assigned to an execution priority
queue. They are assigned a priority by a call to the resident
subroutine PRIOR which is included as one of the first execu-
table statements in the program. The nominal availability of
the primary signals and the normal/acute/wait information is
obtained from digital inputs controlled by an array of switches
at the bedside (the "status panel"). FUZ1 first reads the
state of the switches into an array, S, through a call to DIGIN,
with the bed number and the array name as parameters.
(Table II lists the calling parameters of all of the systems
subroutines for reference through this section.) If it is determined that the "wait" button is on, the program exits after
calling a subroutine DISAST, which, through a call to the
system subroutine CCIWR, writes asterisks after the values
of the variables on the status display indicating that they are
not current. If "wait" is not on, any asterisks previously
written are erased.

```
 1          SUBROUTINE FUZ1 (NBED, IDUM)
 2          IMPLICIT INTEGER (A-Z)
 3          DIMENSION S(13), BUFF(5), IG1(6), IG2(3)
 4          EQUIVALENCE (ACUTE, S(2)), (WAIT, S(3)), (AP, S(4)), (VP, S(5))
 5          EQUIVALENCE (IG2, FG2), (MZ, ZM), (HR, S(6))
 6          REAL FG2(3)
 7          REAL ZM
 8          LOGICAL ACUTE, WAIT, AP, VP, HR
 9          DATA MZ /-1073741824/
10          DATA IG1/'HR ', 'STAT1', 'STAT2'/
11          IBED=NBED
12          CALL PRIOR (2)
13          NP=10
14          LOCCT=0
15          CALL DIGIN(IBED, S)
16          IF (WAIT) GO TO 7
17          CALL DISAST(IBED, 1)
18          IF (HR) GO TO 20
19          IF (AP . OR. VP) GO TO 30
20          FG2(1)=ZM
21          FG2(2)=99999. 0
22          FG2(3)=99999. 0
23          GO TO 46
24   7      CONTINUE
25          CALL DISAST (IBED, 2)
26          GO TO 90
27   20     CALL TIME (1, MOM)
28          IT=KHANF (IBED, 11)
29          CALL ANA(10, 10, II, 1, 1, IT, BUFF, 2)
30          CTACH=0
31          DO 1000 J=1, NP
32          CTACH=CTACH+I2F(BUFF, J)
33   1000   CONTINUE
34          CTACH=CTACH*24/16384
35          IF(CTACH . GT. 150 . OR. CTACH . LT. 35) GO TO 65
36   30     IF(ACUTE) GO TO 35
37          MOML=9
38          CALL GETDAT(IBED, 'HEMO', MOML, 1, IG1,IG2, IC, &35, LOCCT)
39          IHR=FG2(1)
40          IF(. NOT. HR . OR. FG2(1) . EQ. ZM) GO TO 60
41          IF(IABS(IHR-CTACH). GT. IHR/10) GO TO 65
42   60     IF(MOM-MOML . GE. 5) GO TO 70
43          GO TO 90
44   35     IF (AP . OR. VP) GO TO 70
45   45     FG2(1)=CTACH
46          FG2(2)=99996.0
47          FG2(3)=99966.0
48   46     CALL TIME (1, MOM)
49          CALL PUTDAT(IBED, 'HEMO', MOM, 3, IG1, IG2, IC, &90)
50          GO TO 90
51   65     CONTINUE
52          CALL DIGOUT(IBED, 5, 1)
53          CALL DELAY (1)
54          CALL DIGOUT (IBED, 5, 0)
55   70     CALL PINIT (IBED, 'TIMO', 0, MOM)
56          CALL PINIT (IBED, 'HEMO', 0, CTACH)
57   90     RETURN
```

Fig. 10. Listing of trigger program for hemodynamic
calculations.

When ECG is available the heart rate is determined
directly by reading the cardiotachometer output of the ECG
preprocessor (Fig. 10, line 29). System subroutine ANA is
used to obtain analog input. It stores the necessary information into a table used by the analog scheduler and optionally
returns control to the application program as a function of the
return parameter. If this parameter is a +1, ANA will fill
the buffer specified with the number of points requested while
allowing other programs to execute. If the parameter is
negative, ANA will start to fill a buffer equal to the size of
the parameter and return control to the application program
immediately to allow processing of the data. Where large
volumes of digitized data are to be retained, it is possible
for the program to essentially double buffer this data and
write it out on the disc. The analog scheduler is triggered
by a clock interrupt (presently set at 500 times per second),
and the interval parameter specifies the number of five
hundredths of a second between analog reads (see Table II).
If the preprocessor indicated a heart rate of less than 35 or
greater than 150 beats per minute, an alarm would be sounded
in the ward, using a sequence of calls to DIGOUT (digital
output) and DELAY. Then HEMO would be scheduled by a
call to PST. If "acute" is on, the logical array is checked
further and if at least one primary signal is available, HEMO
is started by the system subroutine PST and the trigger program exits (Fig. 10, line 56). Subroutine PST is used to
schedule other programs from applications programs in
execution. The calling sequence includes the bed to be associated with the scheduled program, the name of the scheduled

program, the desired interval between executions, and a
parameter through which data may be passed to the scheduled
program. A positive value for the execution interval represents that interval in seconds. A value of zero specifies that
the scheduled program is to be run only once. A characteristic
interval is stored with each program in the library and that
value is specified by a -1 in the interval parameter.

If no primary signals are available according to the
status panel appropriate codes are stored in a hemodynamic
summary of the list-structured patient file. (Figure 11 shows
some of the summaries in a typical patient file, as represented
in the hard-copy output.) To determine the presence and location of information in the patient file, each file contains an
outline which is separate from, but descriptive of, the file.
This serves as a unique table of contents for the particular
patient's data. The headings in the outline are the names of
the summaries. The subheadings comprise the names of the
individual items to be stored in the file under that summary.
Data storage is accomplished by a call to the subroutine
PUTDAT (Fig. 10, line 49). Symbolic labels for the items to
be stored are contained in an array which is an argument in
the call, as is the array of corresponding values. The time
of day, another parameter, serves as a sequencing element
in each summary.

If the "acute" button were not on (line 36), indicating
5-minute monitoring, the most recent hemodynamic summary
would be retrieved from the patient file through a call to
GETDAT. The parameters in the call to GETDAT are all

```
PATIENT # 1057    BED 1  *******    PATIENT # 1057    BED 1  *******

********                            ********

HEMODYNAMIC TIME 14/0530            HEMODYNAMIC TIME 14/0544

ARTERIAL PRESSURE (MMHG)            ARTERIAL PRESSURE (MMHG)
   SYSTOLIC         75                 SYSTOLIC         91
   MEAN             65                 MEAN             69
   DIASTOLIC        59                 DIASTOLIC        58
   DELTA SYSTOLIC    5                 DELTA SYSTOLIC    9
   MAXIMUM DP/DT    -0                 MAXIMUM DP/DT    -0
   MEAN DP/DT       -0                 MEAN DP/DT       -0
   PULSE DEFICIT     0                 PULSE DEFICIT     0

VENOUS PRESSURE (MMHG)              VENOUS PRESSURE (MMHG)
   MEAN             13                 MEAN              6
   DELTA RESP       -0                 DELTA RESP       -0

PULMONARY ART PRESSURE (MMHG)       PULMONARY ART PRESSURE (MMHG)
   SYSTOLIC         -0                 SYSTOLIC         -0
   MEAN             -0                 MEAN             -0
   DIASTOLIC        -0                 DIASTOLIC        -0

ELECTROCARDIOGRAM                   ELECTROCARDIOGRAM
   HEART RATE              97          HEART RATE             109
   MAX R-TO-R INTERVAL     64          MAX R-TO-R INTERVAL     57
   MIN R-TO-R INTERVAL     62          MIN R-TO-R INTERVAL     55
   SD OF R-TO-R INTERVALS  0.0         SD OF R-TO-R INTERVALS  0.0

RESPIRATION RATE  16                RESPIRATION RATE  17

********                            ********

TEMPERATURE (DEG C) TIME 14/0530    TEMPERATURE (DEG C) TIME 14/0540
   RECTAL          36.5                RECTAL          36.5
   LEFT TOE        31.9                LEFT TOE        32.2
   RIGHT TOE       22.9                RIGHT TOE       22.8
   AMBIENT         22.7                AMBIENT         22.6

********                            ********

URINE OUTPUT (ML) TIME 14/0531      URINE OUTPUT (ML) TIME 14/0546
   TOTAL OUTPUT   363.4                TOTAL OUTPUT   365.4
   LAST 5 MIN        .7                LAST 5 MIN        .6
   LAST 60 MIN     30.3                LAST 60 MIN     17.5

********

CARDIAC OUTPUT TIME 14/0526

   CARDIAC OUTPUT L/MIN      3.41
   BODY SURFACE AREA MSQ     2
   CARDIAC INDEX L/MIN/M     2.09
   APPEARANCE TIME SEC       8
   MEAN CIRC TIME SEC        21
   CENTRAL BLOOD VOLUME ML         1
   STROKE VOLUME ML          35
   HEART WORK KGM/MIN        2640
   RES 1 (MAP-CVP)/CO        1597
   RES 2   MAP/CO            1339
```

Fig. 11. Hardcopy output of a portion of the patient file showing the elements contained in the hemodynamic, temperature, urine output, and cardiac output data summaries.

analogous to those in PUTDAT, except time. This parameter
may be an actual time of day, in which case the values of the
most proximate instance of a summary are returned. Or it
may be a code requesting an instance of a summary by its
position in the file (e. g. , the first, last, previous, or next
instance).

The current time of day, obtained by a call to the
subroutine TIME, is used to calculate the elapsed time since
the last HEMO instance. If this were greater than or equal
to 5 minutes, the hemodynamic program would be scheduled;
otherwise, FUZ1 exits.

Just prior to starting HEMO, the trigger program
also starts a time-code output program, TIMO. Using calls
to TIME, DIGOUT, and DELAY, this program generates a
series of variable-width pulses representing the binary coded
decimal 24-hour time. This signal is recorded on a multi-
channel analog tape recorder along with the primary physiological signals.

HEMO proceeds as shown in Fig. 12. The status
panel is checked and the appropriate analog channels to be
read are determined by reference to the bed number parameter
with which the program was started. A call to DIGOUT, with
a bed and line number, turns on a light at the bedside indicating the signal being monitored. The arterial pressure signal
and the R-wave trigger output of the ECG preprocessor are
sampled simultaneously for 10 seconds at the rate of 100
samples per second (the R-wave trigger generates a pulse
corresponding to each heart beat found in the ECG signal).
Data acquisition is accomplished by a single call to ANA which

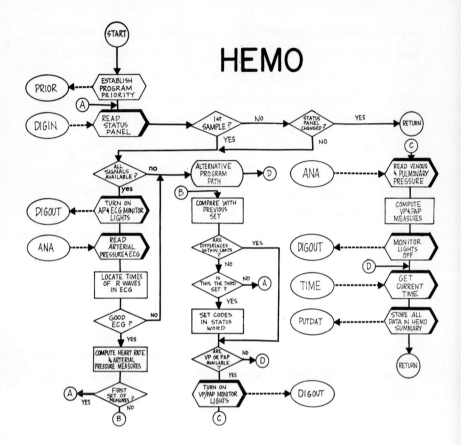

Fig. 12. Flow diagram of the program which performs
the analysis of the pressure and ECG data.

stores 2000 digitized points as 16-bit numbers (half words) in
the assigned buffer.   On completion of the A/D conversion a
second call to DIGOUT extinguishes the channel indicator light.
The array containing the digitized ECG data is then scanned
to locate the heart beats, the relative positions of which are
stored in a table.   The inability to detect a sufficient number
of them in the 10-second sample, or the presence of excessive

noise in the ECG signal, causes the program to take an alternative path. Assuming a good ECG, the arterial pressure
data points are then scanned with reference to the R-wave
table. The maximum and minimum arterial pressure values
detected between each pair of corresponding heart beats are
stored. Anomalous arterial pulse beats are located on the
basis of pulse height criteria, and transient values which
exceed physiological limits are eliminated. The remaining
maxima and minima are averaged and temporarily stored as
systolic and diastolic pressures. Valid arterial pressure
data are scanned to yield maximum and average dp/dt, important measures of cardiac function. The entire arterial pressure data array is averaged to compute the mean arterial
pressure. The maximum, minimum, average, and standard
deviation of the intervals between heart beats is computed
from the R-wave table. Then DIGIN is called again to read the
"status panel." If any switch positions have been changed the
program exits. Otherwise, an additional 10-second sample
of AP and ECG is read and analyzed as above. The results
of the two analyses are then compared; if the differences fall
within preset limits the second set of data is retained and the
program continues. Comparison is performed between the
second and third sets and the new data are either accepted as
consistent or, ultimately, are stored in the patient file with
a code indicating the inconsistency of the sequential samples.
Venous and pulmonary-arterial pressure signals are then
sampled by another call to ANA. From these data, mean
venous pressure, average venous pulse height, and systolic,
diastolic, and mean pulmonary arterial pressure are computed.

TABLE III

Characteristics of Select Applications Programs

Program name	Function	Devices/facilities used	Primary input signals	Data sampling rate (samples/ seconds)	Execution interval (minutes)	Derived variables
1 FUZ1	Schedules execution of HEMO	Patient file system (PFS), digital input (DI), digital output (DO), analog input (AI), program initiation (PI)	Cardiotacho-meter	50	1	
2 HEMO	Monitors hemo-dynamic signals	PFS, DI, DO, AI	Arterial pressure, venous pressure, pulmonary artery pressure, ECG	100	1-5	Systolic, diastolic, mean arterial, mean venous, and mean pulmonary artery pressures, heart rate, pulse deficits, heart rhythm, dp/dt, etc.
3 TEMP	Monitors patient temperatures	PFS, DI, AI	Thermistors	10	5	Rectal, left and right toe, and ambient temperature
4 URIN	Monitors urine output	PFS, AI, DI, DO	Collector tube fluid column height	10	5	Total output, output/ 5 minutes, output/60 minutes
5 PLT2	Writes eight variable time-trend plots on storage scopes	Keyboard/display (K/D), PFS, AO, DO			Demand	
6 MENU	Displays highest level list of user options	K/D, PI			Demand	

	Name	Description	Inputs	Device		Type	Outputs
7	HEDS	Displays hemo-dynamic variables	K/D, PFS				
8	DFIL	Generates line-printer listing of a patient file	PFS, line-printer				
9	CARD	Monitoring and calculation for cardiac output procedure	K/D, AI, AO, DI, DO, PI, PFS, storage scope, ext. interrupts	Densitometer	10	Demand	Cardiac output, stroke volume, central blood volume, peripheral resistance, heart work appearance time, mean circulation time
10	LACT	Determination of blood lactate	K/D, PFS, TTY, PI	Laboratory determination entered through K/D		Demand	Lactate
11	PUMP	Automatic control of pump operation	K/D, DI, DO, AO, PI, PFS			Demand	

Throughout the program the values are checked to see if they lie within reasonable boundaries. If not, or if the primary signal associated with that variable were unavailable, a value of -0.0 is assigned and an appropriate missing value code is stored in a status word. All of the data, including the status word, are stored in the patient file associated with the bed number. The array of data is stored by a single call to PUTDAT, as an instance of the summary named HEMO, identified by the current time of day.

E. Summary

The HEMO program is one of 56 application programs currently in the library. It is representative of the complexity of processing required in patient monitoring programs. Some examples of other applications programs and their characteristics are shown in Table III.

An additional dimension of complexity is contributed by the requirement of simultaneous monitoring of more than one bed. Thus several programs such as HEMO may be in various stages of execution concurrently. Some of these programs may be executed on a scheduled basis while others are executed on request of the clinical staff, making it difficult to predict the demands to be placed on any subsystem of the computer. Simultaneous collection of data from many analog devices, storage and retrieval of data from patient files, and display of critical patient-status information on a variety of devices with varying transmission rates is a common occurrence. Some of these tasks can be deferred or delayed in their execution, but others with crucial responsibilities, such as controlling the infusion of fluids and medications, cannot tolerate interference and may be required at any time.

ACKNOWLEDGMENTS

The research programs of the Shock Research Unit are supported by grants from The John A. Hartford Foundations, Inc., New York, and by the United States Public Health Service research grants HE 05570 and GM 16462 from the National Heart Institute and grant HS 00238 from the National Center for Health Services Research and Development.

REFERENCES

1. Comm. for Admin. Services in Hospitals (C. A. S. H.), Internal Rept. C. A. S. H., Los Angeles, California.

2. J. C. Haldeman, Elements of Progressive Patient Care, Public Health Serv., U.S. Dept. of Health, Education, and Welfare, Washington, D.C., 1959.

3. L. E. Weeks and J. R. Griffith, Progressive Patient Care: An Anthology, Univ. of Michigan Press, Ann Arbor, Michigan, 1964.

4. Hospital Relations Commission, I. C. U. Survey, Hosp. Council of Southern California, June, 1966.

5. H. P. Rome, W. M. Swenson, P. Mataya, C. E. McCarthy, J. S. Pearson, F. R. Keating, Jr., and S. R. Hathaway, "Symposium on Automation Technics in Personality Assessment," Proc. Staff Meetings Mayo Clinic, 37, 61 (1962).

6. J. R. Baruch, "Hospital Automation via Computer Time-Sharing," Comp. Biomed. Res., 2, 291 (1969).

7. L. A. Geddes, H. E. Hoff, C. Vallbona, G. Harrison, W. A. Spencer, and J. Carrzoneri, "Numerical Indication of Indirect Systolic Blood Pressure, Heart Rate and Respiration Rate," Anesthesiology, 25, 861 (1964).

8. R. Smith and W. H. Biddey, The Measurement of Blood
    Pressure in the Human Body, Technol. Survey, NASA,
    Washington, D. C. , April 1964.

9. M. H. Weil, H. Shubin, and L. Rosoff, "Fluid Repletion
    in Circulatory Shock: Central Venous Pressure and
    Other Practical Guides, " J. Amer. Med. Assoc. , 192,
    668 (1965).

10. H. H. Hara and J. W. Belville, "On-Line Computation
    of Cardiac Output from Dye Dilution Curves, " Circulation
    Res. , 12, 379 (1963).

11. H. R. Warner, H. J. C. Swan, D. C. Connolly, R. G.
    Thompkins, and E. H. Wood, "Quantitation of Beat-to-
    Beat Changes in Stroke Volume from the Aortic Pulse
    Contour in Man, " J. Appl. Physiol. , 5, 495 (1953).

12. A. C. Guyton, C. A. Farish, and J. B. Abernathy,
    "A Continuous Cardiac Output Recorder Emphasizing the
    Fick Principle, " Circulation Res. , 7, 661 (1959).

13. B. G. Lamson, "Computer Assisted Data Processing in
    Laboratory Medicine, " Comp. Biomed. Res. , 1, 353
    (1965).

14. D. H. Lindberg, "Electronic Retrieval of Clinical Data, "
    J. Med. Educ. , 40, 753 (1965).

15. W. A. Turner and B. G. Lamson, "Automatic Data
    Processing in Hospitals: a Powerful New Tool for Clinical
    Research, " Hospitals, 38, 87 (1964).

16. S. A. Wilber and U. S. Derrick, "Patient Monitoring and
    Anesthetic Management, " J. Amer. Med. Assoc. , 191,
    893 (1965).

17. M. H. Weil, H. Shubin, and W. M. Rand, "Experience
    with the Use of a Digital Computer for the Study and
    Improved Management of the Critically Ill, " J. Amer.
    Med. Assoc. , 198, 147 (1966).

18. M. A. Rockwell, H. Shubin, M. H. Weil, and P. F.
    Meagher, "Shock III: A Computer System as an Aid in
    the Management of Critically Ill Patients, " Commun.
    ACM, 9, 355 (1966).

19. R. E. Jensen, H. Shubin, P. F. Meagher, and M. H. Weil, "On-Line Computer Monitoring of the Seriously Ill Patient," Med. Biol. Eng., 4, 265 (1966).

20. P. F. Meagher, R. E. Jensen, M. H. Weil, and H. Shubin, "Measurement of Respiration Rate from Central Venous Pressure in the Critically Ill Patient, " IEEE Trans. Bio-Med. Electron., 13, 54 (1966).

21. P. F. Meagher, R. E. Jensen, M. G. Pearcy, M. H. Weil, and H. Shubin, "Automatic Urinometer for On-Line Monitoring of Patients with Circulatory Shock, " Med. Res. Eng., 5, 38 (1966).

22. M. H. Weil, "Computer Automation of Hospitals: Guest Editorial, " J. Amer. Hosp. Assoc., 40, 71 (1966).

23. Roy W. Martin, Automatic Calibration Blood Pressure Amplifier, Proceedings of Eighth International Conference on Medical and Biological Engineering, Section 13-5, Chicago, Illinois, 1969.

24. D. H. Stewart, D. H. Erbeck, and H. Shubin, "Computer System for Real-Time Monitoring and Management of the Critically Ill," AFIPS Conference Proceedings, 33, (December 1968).

25. J. P. Singer, "Computer Based Hospital Information Systems, " Datamation (May 1969).

26. D. H. Stewart and N. Palley, "Monitoring and Real-Time Evaluation of the Critically Ill, " Invited Paper: Journees Internationales d'Informatique Medicale, Toulouse, France, March, 1970.

27. H. Shubin, M. H. Weil, and M. A. Rockwell, "Automated Measurement of Arterial Pressure in Patients By Use of a Digital Computer, " Med. Biol. Eng., 5, 361 (1967).

28. H. Shubin, M. H. Weil, and M. A. Rockwell, "Automated Measurement of Cardiac Output in Patients By Use of a Digital Computer, " Med. Biol. Eng., 5, 353 (1967).

12

Retrospect and Overview

George A. Bekey
Professor of Electrical and Biomedical Engineering
University of Southern California
Los Angeles, California

I. INTRODUCTION

In any fast moving dynamic field, such as the application
of computers to the automation of information flow in modern
hospitals, it is dangerous to attempt to forecast the future.
Therefore, in this concluding chapter we only attempt to
summarize some of the problem areas and to highlight some
of the major themes which recur throughout the preceding
chapters. Rather than to forecast the future, we will attempt
to pose a few questions based on these themes. While there
are many trends which may influence the future development
of hospital information systems, their relative importance is
difficult to assess at the present time. Nevertheless, planning
for a new system requires answers to certain fundamental
questions which emerge from past experience.

II. COSTS

Hospital information systems are sometimes presented
as a panacea for solving the problem of rapidly increasing
costs of hospitalization. However, the experience gained in

many of the systems presented in this book indicates that, at
least initially, hospital information systems must be considered
as an additional cost item for the hospital, adding from $2.00
to perhaps $10.00 per patient day to the cost of hospitalization.
However, once these hospital information systems become
accepted and standard hospital procedures are adopted, there
is a large potential cost saving. A properly installed system
would have sufficient size and capacity to handle a larger
patient population than the one presently under care of the
hospital, so that increases in the number of beds, outpatients,
clinical tests, or other services can be accommodated without additional expense for computer hardware within the
system. Even the software costs may be minimal or nil, if
the system is carefully planned.

One of the major reasons for the possible increase in
cost arising from the introduction of an automated hospital
information system is that in many hospitals the new
computerized system is simply superimposed on top of the
existing manual structure, rather than replacing it. There
are of course excellent reasons for introducing an automated
system gradually. However, in many instances the potential
cost savings of automated systems are never realized, simply
because to realize them would require staff reductions and
reorganizations. A combination of personnel policies,
humanitarian reasons, and timidity on the part of hospital
administrators has sometimes resulted in attempts to keep
the manpower levels constant, thus frustrating any hope for
cost reduction.

The simple truth is that cost reduction from hospital
information systems can only be obtained in two ways:
through manpower reduction, and through capacity for growth
without manpower increases. The growth factor applies both
to increases in patient population which can be handled by the

system, and to the increases in number of patients which can
be handled per unit time through automated procedures.

III. QUALITY OF MEDICAL CARE

The ultimate justification for technological changes within the hospital that do not result in immediate cost savings
must lie in their present or potential capability for improving
the quality of medical care. Yet, perhaps no single factor
is as elusive or difficult to validate as the influence of
automated systems on the quality of health care. In Chapter
5 an attempt to measure the effect of an information system
on this crucial area is presented and it is evident that careful
scientific studies for evaluating health care quality are
difficult at best. It is certainly possible to quantify such
factors as the percentage of a nurse's time spent at the bedside. However, even this factor has only an indirect effect
on the overall result of improved care for the patient. A
proper assessment would require that experiments be designed in which large groups of carefully matched patients in
carefully selected matched hospital settings are treated, using
control group hospitals with manual information systems and
experimental hospitals with automated systems. It is evident
that such studies would be not only difficult, but expensive
and controversial. We must therefore be satisfied with a
number of indirect measures and with the realization that
automated systems provide us with a number of indirect
benefits, such as improved recording of patient data and
history, nearly instantaneous access to patient files, much
greater physician convenience in reviewing patient records,
reduced number of errors in patient files, and a data base
for clinical research.

IV. HARDWARE INFLUENCES

It is evident from even a casual perusal of a number of
chapters in this volume, but there is a great diversity in the
hardware utilized in the implementation of present day
hospital information systems. The computers themselves
range from small, dedicated minicomputers used in the
clinical laboratory to large regional super-computers which
may service a number of hospitals. Communication between
staff and system may take place using teletypewriters,
cathode-ray tube systems, light pen inputs, graphical input
and output devices, and so forth. A large variety of terminals
have been designed for the use of both medical and paramedical personnel, requiring a variety of levels of sophistication on the part of the user. While the hardware trends
are not clearly distinguishable, some major aspects emerge:

1.   There will probably continue to be a trend
      toward the development of large centralized
      regional multi-hospital systems. Each
      individual subscribing hospital would be
      connected with the large computer by means
      of telephone lines, microwave links, optical
      links or some combination of them. The
      advantages of such regional organizations
      are that each individual member hospital
      need not be directly involved in the operation
      and maintenance of the computer center,
      and that costs of operation can be shared
      by member hospitals.

2.   There will probably continue to be a trend
      toward the use of minicomputers in such
      activities as the intensive care unit, the

multi-test screening center, or the
clinical laboratory. Ideally, such
computers will be integrated into the
overall hospital information system.
Within the last few years the costs of
minicomputers have been dropping
rapidly, and it is expected that this
trend will continue in the foreseeable
future.

3.   Terminal devices, providing the interface between the system and the user,
are in a phase of rapid change as well.
We expect that there will be a continuing
trend toward the development of devices
which make it possible to communicate
with the system in natural language and
with a minimum of technical skill. We
expect that complex coding, manipulation
of a large number of control devices,
and even extensive typewriting will
gradually be replaced by the use of light
pens and graphical systems and systems
employing optical character recognition.

V. HUMAN CONSIDERATIONS

It is probably fair to say that no hospital information
system has succeeded in any hospital without the enthusiastic
support of a group of dedicated physicians and other staff
members, who are committed to the automated system. The
use of the automated system spreads by contagion, and the
rate of spreading appears to be directly related to the number

of committed and enthusiastic members of the staff. Here
the cooperation of the medical and administrative staff, the
attitudes of physicians, nurses, technicians, pharmacists
and other members of the staff are absolutely essential. It
is evident that the human factor involved in the acceptance
of new automated equipment is strongly related to the particular hardware interface selected in the implementation of the
system. The more natural, convenient, easy, and time-
saving the system is, the faster will be its acceptance on the
part of the professional staff. Where the automated system
represents simply additional drugery for the convenience of
the business office, the system may go largely unused.
Where it succeeds, it is because it provides not only convenience, improved reporting, and time-savings; but in addition,
a somewhat intangible factor of excitement with the possibilities of the new technology as a tool to aid medicine.
Excitement and enthusiasm are difficult factors to quantify.
Yet, without them, the system may not succeed.

VI. PLANNING FOR HOSPITAL INFORMATION SYSTEMS

It is been emphasized in much of this book that careful
planning is essential if the hospital information system is to
be implemented successfully. In the hospital as in many
other human institutions which have moved toward computer-
based automated systems, a lack of planning may result in
excessive costs, lack of support for the system within the
staff, and ultimate failure. We suggest that as a minimum,
prospective users of new systems should consider the series
of questions presented in the flow chart of Figure 1. While
the order of the questions presented here is not necessarily
crucial, positive answers to all of them probably are. A need

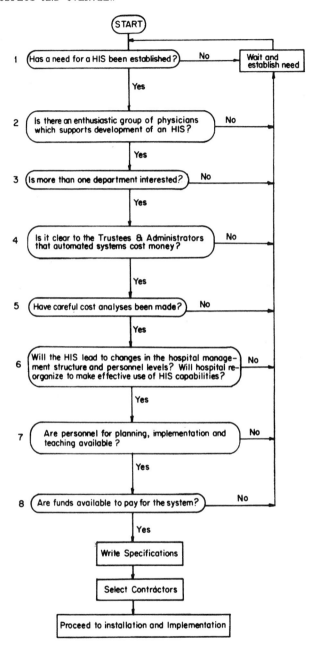

Fig. 1. Planning for H.I.S.

must be established before continuing further. Yet here, at
the very first question, it is evident that no absolute answers
exist. The level of saturation of a manual system, leading
to a need for automated information handling will vary from
hospital to hospital, and must be justified within each individual hospital setting on its own grounds. It is essential
that a dedicated group of both medical and paramedical
personnel exist within the hospital to support the system before any attempts are made to investigate its cost or acquisition. It is essential to ascertain that more than a single
department will be involved in the utilization of the system,
in order to make it cost effective. As indicated above, it is
essential that everyone involved in the procurement of the
system understand the cost implication, and that no one be
deluded into thinking that cost savings will be realized from
the moment that the computer power is turned on. In fact,
cost analyses must be examined with great care, especially
where they involve projections into the future. Based on
past experience it is probably unrealistic to expect that a
hospital information system will pay for itself within the
first two years of operation. If cost savings are expected,
commitments to reduction of staff must be made at the highest
levels and sufficiently early to allow for an orderly transition
from manual to automated procedures. Technical personnel
for implementation of the system should be employed by the
hospital and utilized for such tasks as the writing of specifications and the preparation of new operating procedures,
well before the delivery of the equipment. Finally, only after
positive answers to the above questions have been obtained,
should funds be sought to pay for the system. The final steps,
involving actual procurement and installation, as well as
teaching and follow up can then proceed in an orderly manner.

VII. FINAL NOTE

There is a great variety of hospital procedures.
Physicians are strongly individualistic people, who may be
reluctant to accept rapid or drastic change in their professional procedures. In addition, there is great vitality and
lively competition in the computer industry at the present
time. This combination of factors means that we can probably
expect a continued period of development and experimentation,
as new techniques, new hardware and devices, and new software systems are developed to meet particular situations.
This situation, while leading to uncertainty about the future,
is at the same time an indication of healthy growth. No one
need be deterred from moving into automated systems because they have not yet reached the stage of standardization.
Rather, their active involvement will assist in the acceleration
of the technology as well as in the ultimate goal of improving
patient care at the lowest possible cost. It is evident that
hospital information systems have moved from being a luxury
to being a necessity in the growing progressive modern
hospital. But it is also clear that we have a great deal to
learn and that the last word has not been spoken.

Author Index

Numbers in parentheses are reference numbers and indicate that an author's work is referred to although his name is not cited in the text. Underlined numbers show the page on which the complete reference is listed.

A

Abernathy, J.B., 342(12), 380
Anderson, F., 229(3), 252
Ausman, R.K., 16(29), 35
Azarnoff, D.L., 83(20), 109

B

Baer, R.M., 157(3), 187
Balintfy, J.L., 18(38), 36
Ball, M.J., 215, 223(9), 235(9), 253
Banks, J.A., 83(12,15,16), 108
Barnett, G.O., 10(4,5), 13(20), 32, 34
Bartolucci, G., 325(15), 332
Baruch, J.R., 339(6), 379
Beck, W.S., 13(26), 22(26), 35
Belville, J.W., 342(10), 380
Bernstein, L.M., 325(13), 332
Biddey, W.H., 342(8), 380
Biggs, H.G., 229(15), 253
Brecher, George, 19(43), 36
Brewer, D., 11(7), 33
Brown, Q.R., 13(22), 34
Brunjes, S., 75(1), 84(1), 107
Bunting, S.L., 11(7), 33
Burkes, D., 75(2), 84(2), 85(2), 107

C

Cacciapaglia, A., 14(28), 35
Carrzoneri, J., 342(7), 379
Chinefield, H.R., 19(52), 37
Cluff, L.E., 83(21), 109
Collen, M.F., 19(51), 37, 149 (1,2,5), 157(3,4), 167(7), 169(8), 170(8), 187, 188
Connolly, D.C., 342(11), 380
Constandse, W.J., 229(13), 253
Cotlove, E., 11(7), 33, 226(2), 252
Cromwell, D.F., 13(22), 34
Cronkhite, L.W., 18(40), 36

D

Dantzig, G.B., 157(3), 187
Davis, L.F., 149(5), 157(3), 187
Davis, L.S., 169(8), 170(8), 188
Day, H.W., 319(6), 332
DeGroot, Leslie J., 83(22), 109
Derrick, U.S., 343(16), 380
Dominguez, A., 325(14), 332
Draper, P.A., 83(14), 108
Dreifus, L.S., 325(15), 332

Subject Index

A

Admissions, hospital, 10, 63, 125, 143, 317
Analog signals, 299
Anthropometry, 153
Achilles reflex, 155
Arrhythmia, 319, 322
Audiometry, 156
Autoanalyzer, 193, 195, 222, 232 (see Clinical laboratories)
Automated chemistry program, 217 (see Clinical laboratories)
Automated systems, 2, 150, 189, 194, 341
  in the care of the critically ill, 335

B

Bayer University, 23
Beaumont Baptist Hospital, Texas, 27, 43, 47, 58, 62
Beckman Instruments, Inc., 190
Berkeley Scientific Laboratories, 212, 218, 231
BioScience Laboratories, 241
Blood bank, 205
Blood donor registry, 66
Blood pressure, 153, 322, 367
Blood tests, 159, 194
Bolt, Beranek, and Newman, 26
British National Health Service, 83
Business office, 16, 47, 51, 63
  accounts payable, 57, 64
  general ledger, 57

inventory control, 58
payroll, 56, 64

C

Camarillo State Hospital, 25
Cardiac output, 308, 310, 342
Case histories, 70
Case Western Reserve University, 230
Centralized Laboratory, Long Island, 244
Central Pathology Laboratories, Sacramento, 244
Central processing unit (CPU), 75
Chem-Data Systems, 231
Chester Hospital, Dallas, 47
Children's Hospital, Akron, 48
City Hospital, St. Louis, 238
Clin-Data System, 231
Clinical laboratories, 5, 19, 65, 182, 189f
  autoanalyzer, 193, 195, 222, 232
  automated chemistry program, 217
  computers, 204, 212, 215f, 245
  cost considerations, 189, 205
  data processing, 201
  DNA system, 248
Clinical laboratory computers evaluation, 212
  planning, 251

397

Vital capacity, 155

X

X-ray (<u>see</u> Radiology)

Y

Youngstown Hospital, Ohio,
229, 238